Strained and Drained

Strained and Drained

Tools for Overworked Teachers

Connie Hamilton and Dorothy VanderJagt

ROWMAN & LITTLEFIELD
Lanham • Boulder • New York • London

Published by Rowman & Littlefield
An imprint of The Rowman & Littlefield Publishing Group, Inc.
4501 Forbes Boulevard, Suite 200, Lanham, Maryland 20706
www.rowman.com

86-90 Paul Street, London EC2A 4NE, United Kingdom

British Library Cataloguing in Publication Information Available

Library of Congress Cataloging-in-Publication Data Available

ISBN 978-1-4758-6370-3 (cloth : alk. paper) | ISBN 978-1-4758-6371-0 (pbk : alk. paper) | ISBN 978-1-4758-6372-7 (ebook)

∞™ The paper used in this publication meets the minimum requirements of American National Standard for Information Sciences—Permanence of Paper for Printed Library Materials, ANSI/NISO Z39.48-1992.

To frontline educators who selflessly and wholeheartedly provide a safe, nurturing, and quality learning environment. Thank you for your ongoing commitment to tomorrow's future.

Contents

Foreword

Nathan Maynard

The Buddhist spiritual leader, Dalai Lama was once asked what surprised him the most about humanity, he responded with the profound answer "Man! Because he sacrifices his health in order to make money. Then he sacrifices money to recuperate his health. And then he is so anxious about the future that he does not enjoy the present; the result being that he does not live in the present or the future; he lives as if he is never going to die, and then dies having never really lived." I didn't believe or understand this when I was growing up. I spent much of my childhood hearing my hard working grandfather's stories, as an Italian immigrant in America. He taught me to believe that the harder I work—the more success I would have. As a result, my self-care came second to my work. While I still maintain the work ethic my grandfather instilled in me, the Dalai Lama's words remind me that in order to do my best work, I have to have peace and live for today.

Not prioritizing my self-care, quickly led me to what many of us have in education/youth work, *compassion fatigue*. The toll of supporting the social and emotional health of so many others, comes with a cost to our own well-being. In my fourth year working in a residential treatment care center, I started to realize the impact compassion fatigue had on me. My friends stopped calling me back and people avoided hanging out with me. It caused me to self-reflect. I realized my inner voice and my interpersonal communication exposed the compassion fatigue I was facing. I wasn't just "venting" anymore, I unloaded students' stories and the pain I saw that the kids in the criminal justice system were experiencing. Talking to others didn't make me feel any better; I even started to feel worse. I was so absorbed in the challenges my students faced, that I started to lose interest in hobbies that brought me joy. At 24 years old my personal past trauma was constantly triggered. I began to question how I would be able to sustain a career as a youth worker.

My role working with youth in education and the criminal justice system wasn't just employment, it was my heart driven passion. I didn't want to leave or find a new field, but I needed a way to cope. I attended multiple trainings offered by our residential treatment care center. What I learned in these professional learning sessions was mixed. Some were helpful. Some caused me more disregulation. But none of them focused on helping me to be at my emotional best. I anticipated that the charismatic and knowledgeable presenter was going to start out like they all did with the famous mantra, "you can't pour from an empty cup." Well, my cup wasn't just empty—it had holes in the bottom of it!. This time, the message was different. It wasn't focused solely on the students; her message was about how I needed to tend to my own wellness.

This trainer started sharing her story. She told us about how she almost had a divorce, how she lost friends, and wasn't fun to be around anymore. I felt like she was telling *my* story. Then she described this beautiful anecdote of how she has an imaginary folder. In it, she would put all of her stress, anxiety, worries, negative experiences, and stuff them in her folder every day at work. It was as if she were holding them to be retrieved at a moment's notice. She said it was not fun carrying the folder, but we are in the field of working with kids that need us the most—and it wasn't possible for her to let go of her folder—not even for a minute.

Not only did she hold all the pain and stress in her folder, but she never put it down. It was always in her hands. After school, she carried it home. When she was talking to her husband she was still holding her school folder. When she tried to have a fun time with friends, the folder came with her. She needed a break from the folder and so did everyone else in her life. Woah—did I feel seen.

She then told us about a routine that changed everything for her. Her strategy was simple but effective. She started visualizing taking her folder every day and leaving it on a specific street corner halfway through her drive. The first half of her drive—she would vent, embrace the pain, and revisit the contents of her folder. Then when she arrived at what she referred to as the folder's street corner, she pictured herself placing the folder next to a lamp post and proceeding to drive away.

When she got home, she no longer talked about the folder. When her mind wandered back to the folder's contents, she would remind herself that the folder's contents would be retrieved on her morning commute to school. This mental routine changed her life. I was instantly inspired to try it, it sounded so easy. At first, when I tried to leave my folder behind, I had a hard time letting it go. As difficult as it was to keep my distance from my folder every night, I continued this mental practice. Soon, it started to work. I was able to separate myself from the folder and its contents and enjoy my life outside of the treatment center. Now, as a fifteen year veteran in youth work and education—I still practice this mental habit of leaving my folder each night and picking it up the next day. It worked for me.

I believe this strategy worked for me because I knew I needed to make a change in the way my folder was impacting me physically, emotionally, cognitively, socially, and spiritually. This strategy brought me enough relief from the strain and drain of my work that I could focus on my overall wellness and be ready to pick up my folder and serve the kids who needed me. The thing is, we are all so different as humans. We all have such rich tapestries of life events that form us to be who we are.

This folder analogy might not work for someone else the way it did for me. It's not about everyone adopting the same habits or routines. It's about finding something that does work for you and something you are open to try—for you. Connie Hamilton and Dorothy VanderJagt have compiled a variety of strategies to look at the whole teacher dynamically across the board. They created this plethora of resources and guides to help you achieve and maintain a rounded sense of wellness. You might not have found your "folder" strategy yet, but if you are reading this book, you are on your way. Self-care is the most important thing we can do to be our best selves. The Dalai Lama and my grandfather had something in common—they both spoke of the agency in our own lives. Find what works for you, and I strongly believe that this book is one excellent resource to support your journey.

* * *

Nathan Maynard is a youth advocate, educational leader, international speaker/trainer, and restorative practices expert. He is the co-author of the Washington Post bestselling and award-winning *Hacking School Discipline: 9 Ways to Create a Culture of Empathy and Responsibility Using Restorative Justice*. Nathan also is the co-founder of BehaviorFlip, the first restorative behavior management software. Nathan studied Behavioral Neuroscience at Purdue University and has been facilitating restorative practices for over fifteen years. He was awarded "Youth Worker of the Year" through dedicating his time with helping underserved and underprivileged youth involved with the juvenile justice system in Indiana. He was on the founding administration team that opened Purdue University's first high school in 2017, Purdue Polytechnic High School, serving youth in downtown Indianapolis, Indiana. Prior to his four years as a school administrator, he was a youth worker and program director in a youth residential treatment care center.

He is passionate about addressing the school-to-prison pipeline crisis and closing the opportunity gap through implementing trauma-informed behavioral practices. Nathan has expertise in Dialectical Behavioral Coaching,

Motivational Interviewing, Positive Youth Development, Restorative Justice/Practices, and Trauma-Informed building practices to assist with creating positive school climates.

Preface

Why did you want to become a teacher? As a child, Dorothy was asked by her teacher to tutor other students and she enjoyed teaching her classmates. She admired her teachers and wanted to support children just like her teaching role models did. At a young age, Connie was playing school with her stuffed animals as students. Being her stuffed penguin's teacher provided hours of fun. Doing it "for real" was always her dream. Like us, the response to this question comes easily for most educators. We all know what motivated us and would keep us coming back semester after semester. However, the health and wellness of overworked teachers are in jeopardy. If we don't take care of ourselves with the same passion we have for our jobs, the strain and drain of teaching will suck the joy out of education.

THE STRAIN IS REAL

According to the University of Utah Education Policy Center, 85% of teachers cited they wanted to make a difference in the lives of children as the main motivator to spend a career in a classroom (Ni & Rorrer, 2018). The top four responses included in figure P.1 fit within a general theme of caring for children and the joy teaching brings.

Teaching takes time, energy, and an enormous amount of planning to build effective relationships, lessons, and learning environments. The fact that teachers make approximately 1,500 educational decisions a day as they have numerous distractions hurling toward them from all directions (Boogren, 2018) is one illustration of the demands of the job. Those who are called to the role are aware that success will require hard work. Because the draw to education was the intrinsic reward, we can conclude that the effort being a teacher requires is worth it if the payoff results in gratification and a sense of joy.

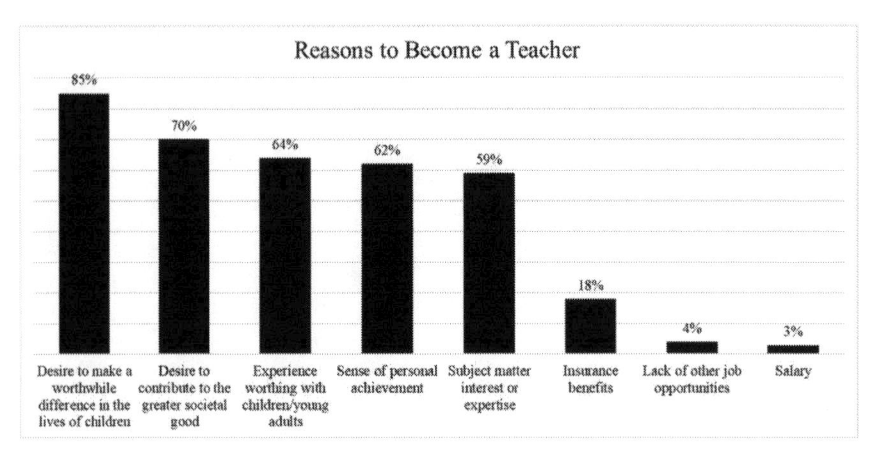

Figure P.1. Reasons to Become a Teacher. The reason 85% of teachers wanted to be a teacher was to make a difference in the lives of children. *Source:* **Ni, Y., & Rorrer, A. K. (2018).** ***Why Do Teachers Choose Teaching and Remain Teaching: Initial Results from the Educator Career and Pathway Survey (ECAPS) for Teachers.*** **Salt Lake City: Utah Education Policy Center.**

Be creative, innovative, and work non-stop. This is the mantra of many teachers. Even when teachers pour more into their work, the workload doesn't seem to lessen. The expectations of educators have grown over the years. The countless hours spent preparing, teaching, assessing, and communicating leaves minimal time to care for their own needs. Teachers are tired and often underappreciated. When this fatigue and criticism set in, levels of stress become harmful.

Burnout is a state of stress that leads to exhaustion, detachment, and feelings of ineffectiveness (Bourg-Carter, 2013). Teachers are burning out at alarming rates. Job stress can lead to depression, anxiety, and insomnia (Greenberg, et al., 2016), and many educators are faced with a heart-breaking decision to endure the strains of teaching or give up their life's' passion.

Dedicated educators find themselves drained physically, emotionally, cognitively, socially, and spiritually. A staggering 61 percent of teachers indicated their jobs were always or often stressful, and more than half of teachers noted poor mental health as a result of that stress (American Federation of Teachers, 2017).

The statistics get worse. A whopping 93 percent of elementary school teachers report experiencing a high stress level (Herman et al., 2018). While teachers are not consistently dealing with life-and-death events within their days, the strain they face daily is real. In fact, teachers and nurses are tied for the most stressful occupation in America today (University of Missouri-Columbia, 2020).

This is not what we signed up for. Teacher wellness is in a state of crisis, and very little has been done systematically to protect our frontline educators.

WHY TEACHERS ARE DRAINED

We might assume that a profession known to produce such a high level of stress would also counteract its effect with equally high coping skills. However, that is not the case. A study that focused on both stress and coping levels found that only 7 percent of all educators reported low levels of stress and high levels of coping skills (Herman, et al., 2018). Without strategies to address the increase in demands, there is little hope to avoid stress and prevent burnout.

The teacher workforce and candidate pool are depleting. The United Nations Educational, Scientific and Cultural Organization reports that 69 million teachers need to be recruited by 2030 to achieve universal primary and secondary education (Coughlan, 2016). Schools all around the United States and the world are scrambling to fill positions. The vacancies in schools place additional demands on the teachers who already work there. Increased class sizes, teaching through prep periods, and supporting uncredentialed teachers who are just getting started in the field punch a direct impact on educators who were already stretched too thin every year.

And speaking of a teacher's year—we would find it hard to believe that there is a single teacher who hasn't heard someone comment about the perceived "cushy" schedule they have. The lack of understanding of a teacher's responsibility leads people to believe that teachers work 32.5 hours, 36 weeks a year, with holidays and summers off. Hmph! Standardized testing, lack of appropriate funding, changing curriculum, new initiatives, state mandates, learning gaps, and policy requirements all impact what teachers have to accommodate annually.

The systemic issues don't even touch the ongoing expectations of lesson planning, assessment analysis, family communication, pupil accounting requirements, material preparation, continuing education, and—should we go on? The point is, the time commitment for the basic function of the job *far* exceeds the contractual minutes teachers are assigned.

As expectations rise, our frontline educators are out of options for how to meet those expectations. The time has to come from somewhere, so every teacher has the unique and painful dilemma of choosing to rob parts of their private lives to fulfill the demands of their job or fall short of the expectations of their job.

Teachers who commit to their roles completely have no other option but to take away from their family or themselves. There simply are not hours and hours floating around waiting to be filled by whatever the demand *au jour* obliges. On the other hand, teachers who draw a line and prioritize their lives outside the school walls are often perceived as undedicated or—as the evaluation tool might label them—unsatisfactory. This conundrum damages the very spirit that led many teachers to dedicate their lives to educating our future.

Sadly, many teachers feel depleted. For those who feel the strain of being overworked, areas of their overall wellness suffer. Late nights grading papers lead to insufficient sleep, lack of empowerment causes feelings of frustration, continuous changes require constant high cognitive demand, insufficient time reduces opportunities for social connections, and the desire to do more than they're capable of evokes internal conflict.

In this situation, not enough teachers pause and put the oxygen mask on themselves. Whether they are unaware of the damage being done to multiple areas of their health or they dismiss the needs their body and mind are craving, the problem overworked teachers face is that some part of their overall wellness is suffering.

Less than 15% of teachers would recommend education as a career choice to others (Owens, 2015). This isn't because they don't enjoy the precious time they have with students. It's everything else the job brings. Intentional care for the well-being of teachers must be a priority.

Some awareness is emerging on the magnitude of the problem. Rather than waiting for a rescue plan to reduce teacher stress, we offer coping options so teachers can take control of their own wellness and make choices that benefit their physical, emotional, cognitive, social, and spiritual health. We believe teachers can still enjoy the pleasures and benefits that helping students learn provides. When properly equipped, we contend that teachers can find a healthy balance that allows them to live a fulfilling life *and* be a quality educator.

A WELLNESS BACKPACK

We know teachers to be giving, dedicated, and caring humans. Unfortunately, these admirable traits are over-extended and contribute to the straining loads teachers are carrying. We see it as if teachers are planning a hiking trip and need equipment to help them navigate the rustic trail of teaching. They need water to stay hydrated, a map or compass to guide their way, a walking stick to keep them balanced on uneven ground, a flashlight to see in the darkness, a tent for shelter, a first-aid kit to nurse injuries, and maybe a camera to capture the beauty of the hike. Imagine trying to juggle all this gear without a backpack. Something has to go.

Teachers are metaphorically carrying heavy loads. When a load cannot be lightened, a better way to carry the load can make all the difference. Backpacks allow loads to be carried longer, and frees your hands. When hiking, your hands might be used to push brush out of your way, maintain your balance, or use equipment like a compass when you need it. For teachers, a wellness backpack frees their hands to *teach*.

With the right strategies and coping skills packed and ready when needed, teachers are better prepared to address the strains and drains on them personally. We want teachers to enjoy the daily hike they take every day when they step into the school building. Whether you feel lost and worried that your supplies are not going to sustain you and feel ill equipped to battle the dangers of the outdoors, or you're ready to take in the joy of nature on a leisurely walk, a carefully equipped backpack can help.

The strategies and ideas shared in *Strained and Drained: Tools for Overworked Teachers* are designed to load your backpack with what you need to not only survive teaching, but to enjoy the journey too.

Introduction

The most recognized definition of wellness comes from the Global Wellness Institute (2021). It defines wellness as "the active pursuit of activities, choices, and lifestyles that lead to a state of holistic health." A close read of this definition draws attention to some key words and phrases. Understanding what wellness means might shift the way you think about it. First, the phrase "active pursuit" suggests that wellness is a process, not a goal we strive to achieve. The goal of wellness is offered in the last part of the definition: "a state of holistic health." The wellness path to well-being and holistic health is paved with the processes of engaging in activities, making choices, and developing habits that form a lifestyle that leads you to better multidimensional health.

According to a study by JBI Library of Systematic Reviews self-care is defined as "the set of activities in which one engages throughout life on a daily basis" (Godfrey et.al, 2010). The clarity of this definition lies in the words "throughout life on a daily basis." What self-care is *not* is an indulgence to make yourself happy in the moment, only to return to a poor state of holistic health. Of course, treating yourself to something is a great way to celebrate you, but do not confuse it with the actions needed to address your personal self-care.

If you chose this book or if it was gifted to you in hopes of generating quick fixes to lift your spirits or easy ways to eliminate the demands of teaching, you won't find it. Instead, we have carefully selected activities and steps you can take to build habits that are likely to improve your overall wellness. You will benefit from a mindset of considering what you need over what you want. Self-care is not always easy and sometimes, it is even unpleasant. But it's necessary.

UNPACKING THE CHAPTERS

There is an intentional text structure that is designed to make it easier for you to get the most out of this book. The first five chapters focus on a specific area of wellness: physical, emotional, mental, social, and spiritual. Then within each of these five chapters, there are sections, each with a distinct purpose. They include, background information, habit building, maintaining your self-care during the school day, options for a quick but temporary boost, suggestions for supporting others, an anecdote of a teacher success story, and tools for your personal needs assessment and action plan. We close the book with chapter 6 where we merge the five areas of wellness to reflect on your wellness holistically.

Our research on teacher wellness uncovered some interesting facts, and some misconceptions. Each chapter opens with background information that defines one of the five areas of wellness. This opening gives you insight to the importance of a specific area of your wellness. When you understand how your daily actions are affecting your overall well-being, you can be more mindful in your choices. Better decisions, although sometimes hard, will benefit you in the long run. Additionally, in this section you will find how neglecting to provide self-care can impact your health.

After some background is provided, the next section looks at ways you can bring specific self-care behaviors into your routine. People who intentionally embed habits of self-care into their lives are more likely to enjoy a life of holistic health. One by one, we isolate the five areas of wellness and offer options to bring them into every one of your days.

Remember, it will be more powerful for you to look at these suggestions based on what you know you need to improve your self-care. Sufficient rest, for example, is included in chapter 1 on physical wellness and self-care. If you already have a bedtime routine and get plenty of sleep, it might make more sense for you to tackle a more urgent physical need and make an effort to establish habits around healthy food choices or increasing your weekly minutes of exercise. It's less about what is fun and easy and more about what will make an impact.

Job-embedded habits and activities are the focus of the next section in the areas of wellness chapters. As educators ourselves, we understand the unique structure of a teacher's "typical" day. Here's a fun fact to prove it: Did you know that in 2016, *Prevention Magazine* cited teachers along with truck drivers and nurses as the occupations that get the most urinary tract infections? Teachers can't even go to the bathroom when they need to.

Because of the extraordinary working conditions teachers face, it's important that self-care not be thrown on a teacher's plate as one more thing they have to do. Or worse, seen as another commitment before or after school when time is already sparse for busy teachers. Therefore, each chapter provides a practical implementation of each of the five wellness areas *within* the school day. Just because you are teaching from bell to bell, doesn't mean your cultivation of self-care halts.

Consistent effort to maximize self-care strategies will help prevent dips in your wellness. For example, if you make a point to enjoy lunch with a close friend every Saturday afternoon, you're less likely to suffer from feelings of isolation. However, even the best plans can get thrown out of whack. We recognize there are times when you can mindfully recognize when your wellness is taking a dip. While we maintain that lifestyle and habit building is the most effective way to maintain a path to overall wellness, there are times when a kick in the pants can give you the boost you need to snap you out of a slump. Therefore, every chapter includes ways to intentionally surge an area of wellness.

As you read through the chapters, you will be encouraged to reflect and assess your level of attention to each of the five areas individually. You may find an area of stability. Everyone's journey to wellness is personal and unique. If your backpack is well equipped with strategies in a certain area of your wellness, we encourage you to preserve the good you're already doing; celebrate your strengths.

Some teachers will be ready to share the contents of their wellness backpacks with others. Maybe you have an established exercise routine and consider yourself fit. You may build on the positive effects that running produces by starting a Run Camp within your school or neighborhood. Each chapter touches on how you can share self-care habits where you excel to use your success and talents for the greater good.

A "Feature the Teacher" vignette is also included in each of the first five chapters. These stories share how an educator tends to self-care or overcame a challenge in one of the five areas of wellness. The celebrations of teachers who are prioritizing their self-care in innovative ways are intended to serve as inspiration to you. As you visit each "Feature the Teacher" section, allow your mind to creatively consider how you might take the necessary steps to put you on a path to holistic wellness.

While some of the anecdotes might attract you on a fun and easy level, others might bring to light the work and effort self-care is. Remember, your journey to relieve the strains and drains that teaching has on you might be challenging at times. Determination to reach an optimal state of well-being will likely require the discipline to choose actions that are good for you, even if they aren't enjoyable.

Each chapter closes with a call to action. Reading about how you can contribute to your well-being is only the first step in building habits of self-care.

To help you develop an action plan, reflection strategies, assessment tools, and planning guides are provided for each area of wellness.

Then, chapter 6 will help you think about how physical, emotional, cognitive, social, and spiritual wellness work together. Since each area is not independent of the other four, the big picture is the only way to avoid sacrificing one area of your wellness to support another. For example, if making and eating breakfast each morning eats up the time you used to spend in quiet thought, you might be robbing a routine that benefits your spiritual wellness to fulfill a physical, nutritional need. This scenario doesn't remove deficiencies; it trades them. To avoid this common flip-flop, the book closes with a view of the whole teacher.

YOUR COMMITMENT TO WELLNESS

Your wellness backpack will be what holds the activities and choices you have that benefit your wellness. The effort you make to mindfully fill your backpack with what you need will prepare you for the journey to holistic health. *Strained and Drained: Tools for Overworked Teachers* will guide you through practical strategies. Some strategies can be implemented immediately, and others will take more careful thought and consideration. This book is not a checklist, but a comprehensive overview of the different areas of self-care that you can use to decide what works for you to integrate and embrace.

Your recognition that a book titled *Strained and Drained: Tools for Overworked Teachers* was worth your precious time is evidence that you are already aware of a need to make changes in your personal and professional life to maintain your well-being. As you embark on this path of prioritizing wellness, be honest with yourself about what you need. It is our hope that you will find something in each chapter that contributes to a decrease in the stress you are experiencing. Wellness is not a destination, it is a way of life. Educating yourself on how you can thrive as a friend, partner, parent, child, sibling, colleague, community member, and teacher is the first step in taking control of your well-being.

Chapter 1

Integration of Physical Well-Being

When you think of physical self-care, you probably first think of exercise. While there is no denying that exercise in the form of cardio has health benefits, there are more factors that affect your overall physical wellness.

Taking care of your sleep habits, feeding your body the nutrients it needs, and protecting your overall health are also contributors to your well-being. Self-care is not limited to a checklist of doing this and you'll feel good. How you feel from day to day can also be impacted negatively by habits you have that are unknowingly harming you physically and keeping you from being at your best. Knowing what to start, stop, and continue doing to bolster your physical care is the first step in improving.

In this chapter, you will read about how sleep, diet, and movement benefit or thwart your physical health. These questions are provided to guide you through the reading. Use them to bring forth what you already know and believe about physical wellness and self-care. At the end of the chapter, reflection questions are provided to assist you with processing the information you read in this chapter.

1. What is my current understanding of physical wellness?
2. In what ways do I think sleep, diet, and movement impact my physical wellness?
3. How do I tend to my physical well-being?
4. What can I do to improve my physical health?
5. What is something I hope to learn as I read?
6. How would I rate my current physical well-being barometer?

THE BRAIN AND BODY CONNECTION

Many of the benefits of being physically active are commonly known. Getting regular exercise lowers the risk of heart disease, helps you maintain a healthy weight, and strengthens your bones and muscles. It doesn't end there. Physical activity doesn't just keep your body fit. According to the American Heart Association, adults who are physically active for a minimum of 150 minutes per week reap benefits of brain health, better sleep, and have fewer symptoms of emotional health risks like depression and anxiety.

While busy teachers are likely aware of the many benefits that exercise provides, finding time can be a challenge. The next section offers ways to make tending to your physical well-being a habit. However, it's important to understand the big picture of physical well-being, and it's not just about exercise. There are other facets of your physical well-being that impact your brain's ability to stay sharp and give you the energy you need in and out of the classroom.

Sleep Is Work

Your body and mind require rest. Sleep allows you to recharge and rejuvenate; more than a third of adults in America are not getting enough sleep (Manella, 2016). Teaching requires mental sharpness and quick response time. Your brain has a job to do when your body is sleeping.

Various sleep cycles are performed when you're resting. Without enough time to sleep, your brain can not process events and information from your waking hours. You may have experienced difficulty retrieving details of the previous day after a restless night's sleep. This is because the brain consolidates information and files it in the brain in places where it makes sense so that you can access the information easily. Lack of sleep prevents this important nightly task from transpiring, which results in delays in your recall.

Another task on your brain's to-do list when you sleep is to adjust hormone levels. The brain takes measures to help keep you asleep so it can get to work. Melatonin is released throughout your slumber, controlling your sleep patterns. In the evening, your melatonin levels increase, making you feel sleepier.

Another interesting fact is the use of antidiuretic hormone (ADH). ADH is released using your body's internal clock. It helps reduce your need to urinate at night, allowing you to have consecutive hours of sleep. A growth hormone, released by your pituitary gland, also gets to work while you're dreaming. Its role is to help your body repair itself.

If you have suffered a paper cut while grading papers, your body works through the night to heal. Cortisol, known as the stress hormone, begins to drop in the first hours of sleep. Before you wake up, the levels rise again. This level of cortisol, after a full night's rest, is what provides us with the refreshed feeling we have when we wake up. It is also the hormone that turns on our appetite, which we will address later in this chapter.

Your immune system gets attention as you sleep, too. Proteins called cytokines are released in small amounts. They fight off inflammation, infection, and trauma if you're sick or injured. Your fight-or-flight response is controlled by your sympathetic nervous system. When you are sleeping, this system gets to take a breather. This is especially helpful in maintaining healthy blood pressure levels which, if not controlled, can cause an increased risk of heart disease.

It might be helpful to think of your body as a 24-hour system. When you are tempted to rob time dedicated to sleep in order to complete more tasks, you are essentially choosing to limit your opportunity to process what you accomplished during the day and denying your body the chance to heal and regulate itself.

The Centers for Disease Control and Prevention's (CDC) recommendation for adults to get a minimum of seven hours of sleep each night is not an arbitrary number. This is the amount of time necessary for the brain to complete its nightly duties. It improves the quality of your life and increases your life expectancy. So ditch the "You can sleep when you die" slogan, because that type of thinking will get you there sooner.

As teachers continue to pack more into each day, the importance of sleep is often underestimated. Teachers are texting, watching videos, and using devices from morning until bedtime. These devices are not helping anyone rest. Electronic devices are affecting your ability to sleep well. Screens emit blue light that suppresses melatonin, the chemical that regulates circadian rhythms, making it difficult to fall asleep and stay asleep (Harvard Health Letter, 2020). Setting limits on technology and keeping a routine are good ways to begin focusing on sleep.

You Are What You Eat

How we talk about a healthy diet has shifted over the years. The guidelines from the United States Department of Agriculture (USDA) were first published in 1894 and have progressed over the years (Jahns et al., 2018). The four basic food groups were introduced in 1956 and their use was recommended for thirty-six years. In 1992, four basic food groups shifted to a food pyramid that added fats, oils, and sweets to the picture.

The most notable change included recommendations for daily servings in each category. However, this hierarchical image was criticized by nutritionists because of the way it suggests that grains should make up the largest portions, without any distinction between healthier food choices within the categories like quinoa versus pasta or popcorn versus potato chips.

Consequently, the pyramid got a facelift in 2005 that removed the suggestion of hierarchy and added a stair climber to reference the need to balance diet and exercise. The primary image was often shared without food and limited information. The USDA encouraged users to personalize their pyramid, which caused a thumbs down by many due to the complexity of its use.

In 2011, First Lady Michelle Obama unveiled MyPlate, the tool used today. MyPlate, shown in Figure 1.1, shows five food groups. The icon shows approximately four cups of fruits and vegetables to fill half the plate. The other half consists of 6 ounces of grains and 5 ½ ounces of protein. A small circle represents the three cups of recommended dairy consumption (USDA, 2021).

There are plenty of resources to help you manage your diet if you're trying to build muscle or lose weight. Eating a balanced diet fuels your body so you have the energy needed to perform without getting tired or risking illness. This information provides general wellness ideas and is not intended as a substitute for professional medical diagnosis or advice. Always consult a medical professional for any changes in your healthcare plan or if you think you have a medical condition.

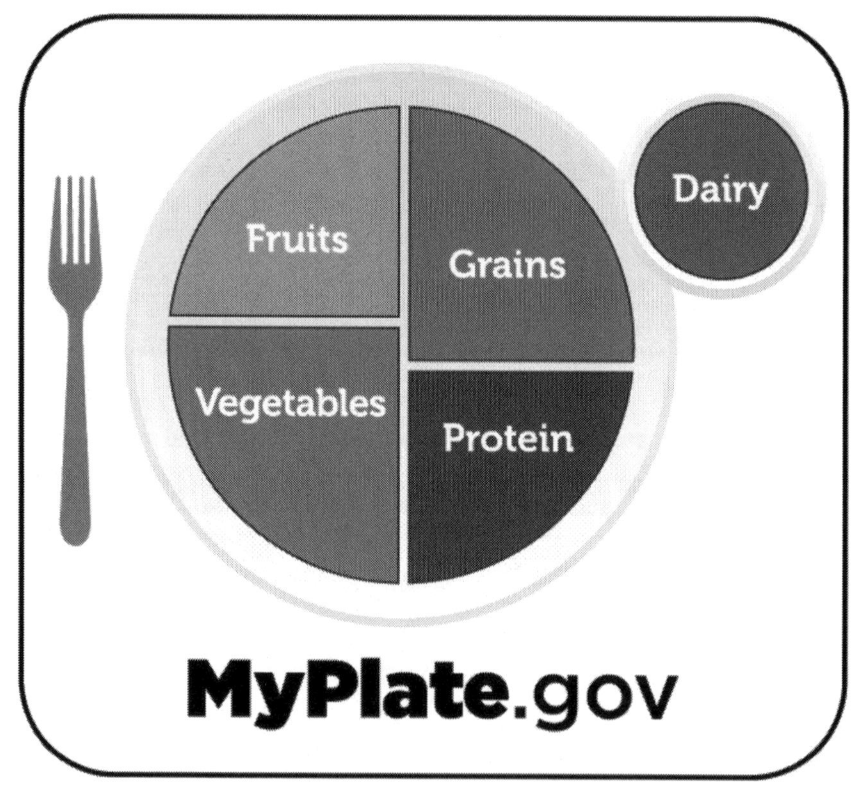

Figure 1.1: My Plate. *Source:* U.S. Department of Agriculture. https://www.myplate.gov/resources/graphics/myplate-graphics

Keep in mind the primary purpose of eating is to fuel your body. Therefore, a mindful selection of foods that offer the nutrients your body needs will help you feel energized and sharp, and stay healthy.

The Joy of Movement

There simply cannot be a chapter about physical well-being without pumping the benefits of exercise. Robin Sharma, the best-selling author, has been known to say, "If you don't make time for exercise, you'll probably have to make time for illness" (as cited in Piercy & Troiano, 2018). Almost 80% of adults and adolescents in the United States are insufficiently active (Piercy et al., 2018). Failure to get enough exercise is linked to a laundry list of problems including difficulty sleeping; poor cardiovascular health; being prone to injury, anxiety, and depression; stress; weakened bones; and premature death.

You might have been told you need to clock 10,000 steps per day. There is actually no magic to this number. This well-known pedometer goal stems from a marketing campaign centered around the 1964 Tokyo Olympic Games. A company sold a pedometer called Manpo-kei: "man" meaning 10,000, "po" meaning steps, and "kei" meaning meter. Its popularity and success made the link between pedometers and 10,000 steps stick. It's so widely used that even step counting apps throw virtual confetti when you take your 10,000th step.

One researcher compared the number of steps women in their seventies took each day with the likelihood they would die from any cause. After an average of four years, women who took 4,000 steps per day were significantly more likely to be alive than women who only walked 2,700 steps. As the number of steps increased, the study did show a decrease in mortality, but there was a limit. After a total of 7,500 steps, the benefits plateaued. So, what does this mean? It means there was no significant evidence that reduced mortality beyond 7,500 steps a day (Lee et al., 2019). Therefore, the magic of 10,000 steps is not supported by science.

The Department of Health and Human Services doesn't make recommendations based on step count. It recommends that adults get 150 minutes of moderate aerobic activity or 75 minutes of vigorous aerobic activity per week (Laskowski, 2021) (see Figure 1.2). You can expect to see immediate results of a good workout in the form of better sleep (National Sleep Foundation, 2013), reduced short-term anxiety, and improved cognitive function (United States Department of Health and Human Services, 2018).

To manage exercise time, people have more success with shorter, more frequent bursts of activity than longer sessions (Angle, 2018). Table 1.1 shows ways you can spread 150 minutes over the course of a week. Option 1 equalizes time five days a week. This is ideal for people who want a weekday routine.

Moderate Intensity
150 minutes per week

You can talk, but can't sing
You are sweating
64-76% your maximum heart rate

- Biking (slower than 10mph)
- Brisk walk (2.5 miles per hour)
- Gardening
- Heavy cleaning (washing windows, vacuuming, mopping)
- Pushing a lawnmower
- Raking leaves
- Stair walking
- Shooting hoops
- Washing or waxing car
- Water aerobics
- Weight Training
- Yoga

Vigorous Intensity
75 minutes per week

You can't talk without pausing
Breathing hard and fast
77-93% your maximum heart rate

- Aerobic dancing
- Circuit weight training
- Cycling 10 mph or faster
- Heavy yard work like digging or hoeing
- Hiking uphill or with heavy backpack
- Jumping rope
- Karate, judo, tae kwon do, jiu jitsu
- Playing basketball or soccer
- Running
- Shoveling snow
- Skiing
- Swimming laps
- Tennis
- Wheeling a wheelchair

Figure 1.2: Moderate and Vigorous Activities. ***Source:*** **Connie Hamilton**

Option four in Table 1.1 is broken into specific exercises and shown in Figure 1.3. Of course, greater amounts of exercise bring additional benefits, but any amount of physical activity you can include in your life is helpful. Pause to think about how much exercise you fit in each week normally, and consider what might be some ways to help you get closer to the 150 minute weekly goal.

GETTING INTO A PHYSICAL GROOVE

The thought of building habits that support your physical well-being can be overwhelming. Many times, our defense mechanisms kick in at even the suggestion to add one more thing to our overworked plates. However, living a

Table 1.1: Weekly Exercise Options

	Mon	Tues	Wed	Thurs	Fri	Sat	Sun
Option 1	30 mins	30 mins	30 mins	30 mins	30 mins	X	X
Option 2	X	50 mins	X	50 mins	X	X	50 mins
Option 3	15 mins	30 mins	15 mins	30 mins	X	60 mins	X
Option 4	15 mins	15 mins	15 mins	15 mins	15 mins	75 mins	X

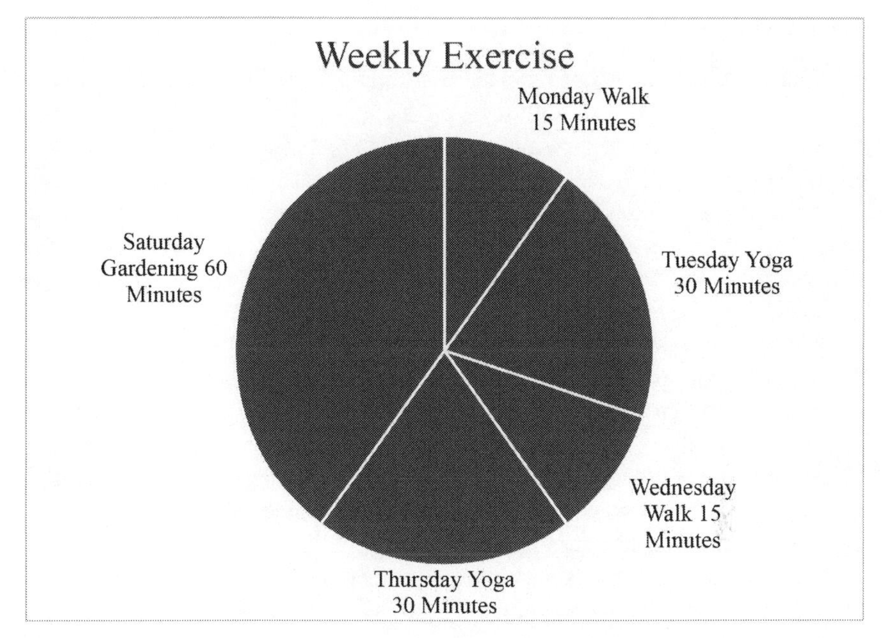

Figure 1.3: Weekly Exercise Chart. ***Source:*** **Connie Hamilton**

life in and out of the classroom that contributes to quality sleep, a healthy diet, and physical activities doesn't have to be a complete upheaval of your current style. Some of the simplest steps you can take (no pun intended) to bring physical self-care into every one of your days are captured in this section.

Stock Your Kitchen

Convenience is an undeniable reason why we choose what we eat. If your refrigerator is packed with soda and frozen pizza, then frozen pizza and soda become an option when determining your meal. If you stock your pantry and kitchen with foods that provide the nutrition you need to care for your body and mind, your options can include grilled chicken and cucumber water.

Other tips from Michael Greger's (2015) book *How Not to Die: Discover the Foods Scientifically Proven to Prevent and Reverse Disease* suggest a "daily dozen" that includes beans, berries and other fruit, cruciferous vegetables such as broccoli and cauliflower, greens and other vegetables, flaxseeds, nuts, whole grains and spices. We know it's hard to resist a buy one, get one free (BOGO) sale on chips. But your instant decision to swap out chips for celery and carrots when you're at the grocery store will impact what you're snacking on all week.

What's Up, Doc?

A major insurance provider reported that only 50 percent of covered clients attend an annual well visit with their physician. About a third only go to the doctor when something is wrong (Vora, 2015). Let's put this in education terms: Not getting a checkup is like not using formative assessments for your students. It's great news if you check in on a student and they're progressing well. However, when a student is experiencing difficulty, educators know that intervention is better than remediation because an intervention can prevent failure. Failing health is not a risk you should take.

Teaming up with a medical professional can provide you with some options to tackle anything you might be dealing with on your own. Trouble sleeping, a dull headache, or digestive issues might not trigger you to call the doctor but are all examples of symptoms you can share at a wellness visit. Your attribution to work stress could very well be the cause of your increase in blood pressure. However, it could be a sign of something more serious and is worth mentioning to your physician.

Your insurance likely covers wellness checks, appointments don't take long, you can be selective when you schedule your visit, and you might even get peace of mind that you "pass" your checkup. If an issue does arise, you'll be grateful you and your doctor can plan how to address any medical needs that might surface in your visit.

Strengthen Willpower

Willpower allows us to forgo short-term desires in order to achieve long-term results (Lino, 2020). It is the inner strength that moves us toward our goals and helps us create lasting positive change. If you are feeling like this is an area of weakness for you, you are not alone. A survey conducted by the American Psychological Association revealed that 27% of those surveyed indicated a lack of willpower as the main factor keeping them from reaching their goals (Cherry, 2020).

You are not doomed if your current level of willpower is low. You are not born with a certain amount of willpower that remains constant throughout your life. Willpower is like a muscle and, when strengthened, can change and increase (Tunikova, 2018). Avoiding temptation actually avoids the use of willpower. When your willpower is not strong, you might find the best way to resist a donut in the staff room is to not go in the staff room. There's little doubt that if you don't engage with a temptation, you're not likely to succumb to it.

It's not always possible to resist the urge for instant gratification. Oftentimes the temptation is unexpected and could not be avoided. In times like these, people who have exercised and built their willpower are better equipped to keep their eye on the long-term prize that would be jeopardized if they cave in the moment.

Roy Baumeister, a psychologist, shares three necessary components for achieving goals; first, you need to establish the motivation and set a goal; second, you need to monitor your behavior toward the goal'; and the third is willpower (American Psychological Association, 2012). As you focus on building your willpower, these strategies may assist you:

Publicize Your Goals

Tell others what you're trying to accomplish. Just knowing that others are aware of your goal increases your motivation to leverage your willpower.

Keep a Food Diary

Logging your food brings mindfulness to what you eat. The level of awareness is often enough to create an ample pause to allow your willpower to kick in. There are many apps that offer quick and easy meal tracking tools.

Provide Self-Encouragement

Every time you say you can't, you're reinforcing your own lack of confidence. Flipping the narrative that replays in your mind reinforces the positive actions you can accomplish with will power. Instead of saying "I can't find 15 minutes a day to walk," try a more encouraging verbiage like, "I'm going to find 15 minutes to walk today."

Set Your Willpower Up

If you activate your willpower when you're grocery shopping, you might have to exercise it for about an hour as you refuse to put unhealthy items in your cart. Otherwise, if you bring those items home, you have to depend on your willpower daily because the temptation is in your cupboard.

Postpone It

If you are trying to break a bad habit and find your willpower is taxed by the idea of completely eliminating something from your life, try a smaller increment. In his book *Willpower: Rediscovering the Greatest Human Strength*, Roy F. Baumeister and John Tierney (2011) suggest that people offer a compromise to themselves by saying "not now, but later." Oftentimes later never comes, and generally the torment of being tempted by something you can not have is lessened with this approach.

Reward Yourself

If you reach a milestone or success, celebrate with something that keeps you focused on your goal. If you lost the weight you were trying to lose, buy a new outfit. Meeting your exercise goal might lead you in the direction of scheduling a deep tissue massage. When you have successfully had seven or more hours of sleep for a week straight, treat yourself to an activity you don't have the time to enjoy as often as you'd like.

Take as Prescribed

If your doctor has prescribed medication to manage your health, there are always directions to outline when and how much to take. Sure, one dose every morning seems like an easy instruction to follow, but half of the time, medicines are not taken as recommended (Brown & Bussell, 2011). The reasons are often rational. They forget, the side effects are unpleasant, they're feeling better and think the medicine is no longer needed, or the opposite—the patient doesn't think the medicine is working at all, so they just stop taking it.

Part of taking care of your physical health includes managing your medical needs. Whether your prescription is preventative, maintenance, or written to cure a temporary illness, if you're tempted to play doctor with your health, resist. A quick call to the physician's office or pharmacy to inquire about side effects or what to do about missed doses will provide you with expert advice for your specific health care needs. Here are some questions to ask your health care professional if you are prescribed medication:

- What is the medication and how does it work?
- Can I stop taking it when I feel better or should I empty the bottle?
- Is there an advantage to taking it in the morning or night?
- What side effects are normal? What side effects should concern me?
- How will I know it's working?
- What if I miss a dose?
- Will this affect over-the-counter medications?

Change Your Light Bulbs

You've heard of ROY-G-BIV that labels the colors of the rainbow. They also combine as light colors to make the white light you see when the sun is shining. Of all the colors of light, blue light is the main type of sunlight. Fluorescent and LED light bulbs also shine blue or "day" light. Evidence is supporting some benefits of blue light such as increased alertness, memory, improved attention span and reaction times, and a more positive mood.

However, there is also a downside. Blue light is a stimulant and has been proven to have a direct impact on sleep (Beaven & Ekstrom, 2013).

Your biological clock helps regulate your circadian rhythm, which follows roughly a 24-hour cycle. Light signals to your body that it's time to be awake and in the evening, melatonin is produced to help you fall and stay asleep (Dimitriu, 2020). While it's true that all light decreases the melatonin your body releases, blue light has even more impact on the circadian rhythm.

If you spend all day in a classroom with fluorescent light, then come home to a space with light-emitting diode (LED) or blue lights, your environment might be contributing to the amount and quality of your sleep. To protect yourself from unnecessary exposure to blue light, use nightlights with red bulbs instead of ceiling lights or lamps as you get ready for bed.

Smart light bulbs offer the flexibility of shining daylight during your waking hours, then shifting to softer lights in the evening. Schedule a routine with Alexa that switches your smart light bulbs away from blue lights so your body can follow its natural circadian rhythm when it's time for dreaming.

Put Your Screens to Bed First

One of the hardest things for people today is to put down their devices. When we hear an email alert, whether it's curiosity or addiction, we often look to see who's sending a message. In chapter 4 the social ramifications that the constant use of phones has on you will be discussed. For your physical well-being, exposure to screens is bad for your eyes and your sleep schedule. It is recommended that exposure to blue light be limited before bed to avoid the delay of melatonin release. Specifically, interactions with bright television, computer, and cell phone screens should be avoided at least thirty minutes before bedtime (Suni, 2020).

As highlighted at the beginning of this chapter, sleep is required for your body to process memories, heal, and rest. Bright light fools the body into thinking it's daytime so it doesn't release the melatonin needed to help you get a good night's rest. If you're having trouble sleeping, it could be because you were recently using your bright device.

Although you might be tempted to pass the time by playing a mindless game on your phone, that will only delay the messaging to your body that it's nighttime. Put your screens down before you prepare for bed as a habit. If you find yourself having trouble sleeping one night, we offer some tips for falling asleep later in this chapter.

Give Caffeine a Cut-Off Time

"Ninety percent of North American adults consume some form of caffeine daily, making it the most widely used psychoactive drug of all time." This fact from a study conducted by *New Scientist* magazine reminds us that caffeine is a drug (Lee, 2017). There is no drug that doesn't have its risks and your morning cup of java is no exception.

The benefits of caffeine consumption are widely known. It helps keep you alert. As caffeine works, messages are sent to the pituitary gland. All the activity caused by the action caffeine instigates in your brain suggests to your pituitary gland that there is an emergency. When the fight or flight is triggered, your senses become more alert. It's a survival mechanism. We experience heightened awareness and a boost of energy the adrenaline offers.

As with any drug, there are negative effects of caffeine use as well. Teachers might not connect the direct impact caffeine has on their sleep habits. The effects of caffeine can stay in your system for five hours or more (Marengo, 2018). Try to cut out the caffeine intake in the evening. If you're a coffee drinker like us, it doesn't help to switch from coffee to a caffeinated soda. This is a perfect time to get in your daily hydration goal and drink more water.

Have a Weekly Workout

People who exercise for 150 minutes at a moderate intensity week after week enjoy health benefits. Not only are you more likely to extend your life expectancy, but you will also be stronger, have less weight gain, and have a lower risk of heart disease, stroke, type 2 diabetes, high blood pressure, dementia and Alzheimer's, and several types of cancer (Piercy & Troiano, 2018).

Prioritizing actions that benefit your health is of utmost importance, no matter how hectic your schedule seems to be at the moment. You must find ways to carve out intervals in your day that work for you. If you feel short on time or cannot commit to a big chunk of time, spread out the activity during the week so the 150 minutes seem manageable. Find an accountability partner to communicate with regarding your progress, then frequently check in with each other regarding the number of minutes you are exercising a day and encourage one another to break a sweat, drink more water, and eat healthily.

Unbreak Your Back

Teaching is literally a pain in the neck. Studies show that teachers complain of shoulder, neck, and back pain. An occupational hazard of teaching is lower back pain. High school teachers are even more likely to suffer from lower back pain than elementary teachers.

This is a good spot to plug in 150 minutes of exercise per week because, in addition to the benefits previously mentioned, teachers who exercised more had fewer complaints of lower back pain (Kebede, et al., 2019). Long periods of standing and sitting, and a "head down" posture when reading, grading, and writing are to blame for the high number of teachers complaining of a sore back (Kebede, et al., 2019).

Increased movement, frequent breaks, and targeted stretching will reduce the soreness in your muscles. Whether it is writing a book or working on lesson plans, there is a need for interventions with back pain and stiffness from sitting for long periods of time at the keyboard. Stand-up desks help tremendously, but another idea in easing the potential back pain is to take short breaks to get the blood flowing and chunk daily exercise throughout the day.

Instead of 60-minute workouts, pause for a 15-minute mini-yoga session or a short but brisk walk with the dog. Task your roommate or partner with helping you to remember to walk away from the screen, even if you are in a flow. When you're focused on a specific task, it's easy to lose track of time, so solicit the assistance of those around you to offer a reminder that it's time to move.

WHEN YOU NEED A PHYSICAL SURGE

You're not going to be at your physical best every day. Knowing how to fuel your body so you can be at your best is critical. When your energy level is low, you're feeling fatigued, or you need to nurse your own health, these short-term options might give the surge you need to get back in the game. If the list triggers a new idea—more power to you!

Power Snack

Nourish your body with nuts, fresh fruits and vegetables, and foods high in vitamins and minerals to combat fatigue and sustain you throughout the day. Your body lets you know when it is sleepy and low on energy. Some go-to foods for a burst of natural energy are bananas, almonds, berries, and eggs. You can have these snacks with you at school for that quick burst. Figure 1.4 suggests foods that benefit specific areas of physical wellness.

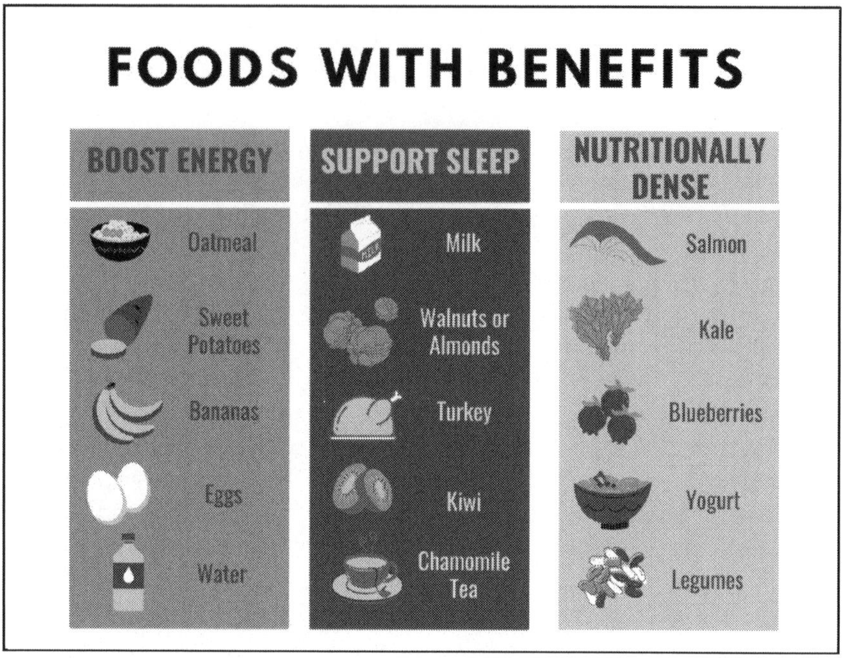

Figure 1.4: Foods with Benefits. *Source:* Connie Hamilton

Make Like a Cat

Cats sleep about two-thirds of every day. When they get tired, then curl up and drift off to sleep. An educator's schedule is unlike a cat's and will not likely find many opportunities to catch some zzzs during instructional hours. Resting late afternoon and before you tend to after-school tasks or taking advantage of a fifteen-minute break on the weekend may be just what you need to give you the boost of energy you're looking for. Just be careful. Napping after 3 pm can interfere with nighttime sleep (Mayo Clinic, 2020), which is necessary for your body and mind to recharge and properly rest.

Reduced number of sleeping hours, excessive stress, poor diet, sedentary lifestyle, and underlying medical conditions all contribute to a feeling of exhaustion (Nichols, 2018). When this happens, teachers, along with other adults, remedy the feeling by trying to get more sleep at night, taking a nap, or reaching for caffeine.

A study conducted in 2008 reported the most effective anecdote before mid-evening was the nap (Horne, et al., 2008). Studies have found that a five-minute doze is too short, but sleeping for more than 30 minutes leaves you feeling groggy when you wake up (Scott, 2020a). The ideal nap is in the

10 to 20-minute range, and these are often referred to as power naps. These power naps help lower stress, and increase learning and efficiency.

As always, consult your physician if you feel you are sleeping more than usual or have trouble staying awake without a logical reason to determine what your needs are or if there is an underlying medical condition.

Maximize Your Java

The authors are not medical experts but wanted to share some more news about napping! Caffeine and napping don't seem like they would work cohesively together, but the research is overwhelming on the subject. Multiple studies, including one shared in 2020, showed that consuming 200 mg of coffee (about 1–2 cups) before taking a 20–30 minute nap allowed nightshift workers who participated in the study to awaken perkier than those who took a placebo.

This "caff-nap" diminished their sense of grogginess and allowed them to show marked improvements in performance and alertness (Centofanti et al., 2020; Schweitzer et al., 2006). The study is not presented as a recommendation, only shared as a reference in case you want to discuss this idea with your doctor.

Strike a Pose

As mentioned previously in this chapter, teachers often suffer from back pain and stretching is one way to counteract the damage that long periods of standing and sitting can do to our bodies. However, stretching also has more generalized benefits.

Stretching increases flexibility, which increases your range of motion and balance. It also increases blood flow and alleviates tension. Improved flexibility helps you perform everyday activities with ease, which is important in your teaching role. Research revealed that a combination of strengthening and stretching muscle groups can encourage proper alignment and reduce musculoskeletal pain (Hotta, et al., 2013).

There are several stretching techniques that help reduce the pain.

Child's Pose

On your hands and knees, sink your hips back and rest them on your hips. Rest your belly on your thighs and keep your hands in front or next to you with your palms up. Breathe and relax for up to 1 minute.

Knee-to-Chest Stretch

Lie on your back with both knees bent. Draw one knee into your chest by pulling on your shin bone to lengthen your spine without lifting your hips. Breathe, hold for one to three minutes, then switch legs.

Piriformis Stretch (Butt Stretch)

Sit in a chair and cross one leg over the knee of the other leg. Keep your back straight and slowly lean forward until you feel a stretch. Hold for 30 seconds and switch.

Inhale, Exhale

There's breathing. And there's *deep* breathing. The list of benefits of various types of deep breathing includes decreasing stress, combatting pain, cleansing the body of toxins, improving immunity, lowering blood pressure, improving digestion, and increasing cardiovascular capacity and energy. We will circle back to some of these benefits in future chapters. Here, we will take a closer look at how deep breathing can give you a needed energy boost.

The stimulating breath has a specific technique. Try it first thing in the morning to trigger the energizing chemical in your brain called epinephrine or more commonly referred to as adrenaline. Here's the basic exercise for the stimulating breath (Rakal, 2016):

1. Sit upright and comfortably.
2. Keep your mouth closed and breathe in and out of your nose as quickly as possible. Your inhale and exhale should be short, deep, and equal in duration. This is not a peaceful, quiet exercise.
3. Try to do a cycle of three breaths in one second. In between each cycle, breathe normally.
4. There is a risk of hyperventilating, so start with fifteen seconds for your first time. Gradually add five seconds at a time until you can exercise your breath for a full minute.

If you have done it correctly, the feeling will be similar to how you feel after a good workout. You will notice your effort at the back of your neck, diaphragm, chest, and abdomen.

Take a Sick Day

When teachers are sick, many weigh the pros/cons of going to school and toughing it out versus tending to their own self-care and staying home. Other factors that flood through a teacher's mind when they're ill include: Do I have enough sick time? How will my principal react? Will the school be able to secure a sub or will my colleagues have to pick up my slack? How will our students stay on track? Do I have enough energy to write detailed lesson plans?

Don't overthink it; if you're sick, stay home. Period. To make the decision to call in a little easier for you, write a sick day lesson plan that is not specific to your curriculum's scope and sequence. When you have pre-arranged absences, there is usually time to make an effort to keep students learning on the current topic. However, when you're unexpectedly under the weather, you'll be thankful for the preparation you made in advance. Some teachers have recorded videos for their sub to play, developed asynchronous lessons, and/or followed established routines to create stand-alone sub plans.

Chillax

An outcome of trying new physical activities might have you using muscles that don't get used very often. You might be sore after a good workout or a long day clearing out the storage room. A warm bath, a heating pad, or a massage is known for reducing pain. These activities are also linked to general relaxation and can help you decompress after a busy day so you will be able to sleep at night. A little personal pampering can reduce muscle tension, helps lower blood pressure, and prevents chronic stress from damaging your health (Scott, 2020b).

"Forget" Your School Bag

If you're like countless educators, you have packed your teacher bag with papers and books with the intent to catch up on schoolwork at home. And, if you're like many teachers, there were nights you lugged that bag right back to the school the next morning without ever opening it. Even though this is totally fine, it's hard not to feel guilty for leaving tasks undone.

If you know you have a busy evening planned with the family, or you want to dedicate after-school hours to tending to your self-care, leave your school bag at school. The temptation to sacrifice your own well-being or necessary sleep time will be removed if you didn't bring the resources home.

Some teachers are able to make this a habit. They regularly finish school jobs in the school building and have a clear separation between their work and personal lives. This is not the norm. Teachers, on average, are at school an additional 90 minutes beyond the school day for various obligations such as: providing after-school help for students, attending staff meetings, collaborating with colleagues, and mentoring others (Bill & Melinda Gates Foundation, 2012).

In 2008, the Bureau of Labor and Statistics reported that teachers are more likely than other professionals to do some work at home (Krantz-Kent, 2008). For the majority of teachers who routinely bring their work home, it can't be said any clearer than this: It's okay to take a night off. There is no prize for the educator who clocks the most hours per week.

BELL-TO-BELL INTEGRATION OF PHYSICAL WELL-BEING

Since most of your waking hours are spent at school, it makes sense to keep your physical well-being in mind when you are teaching. Use moments in the workplace to keep your body active and provide quality food fuel to produce the energy you need to keep up with your students. Here are some ways you can take care of yourself when school is in session:

Walk the Halls

Your school offers the perfect opportunity for you to get some extra steps in. Take the long way to the teachers' lounge or do an extra loop before returning to your classroom. If it's nice outside, take an exit door and walk outside to get to the office.

Schedule Time for Nourishment

Many teachers use their "duty-free" lunch break to make copies, check emails, and prepare for afternoon lessons. Too often, the short time dedicated to consuming a meal is eaten up with these tasks, leaving no time to eat. Teachers need their nourishment! A balanced diet provides your body the nutrients that are critical for it to work effectively. Having a healthy snack drawer in your classroom allows you to select from food choices that promote a robust diet.

Brown Bag It

Sometimes teachers eat what is in the vending machine or completely skip eating lunch altogether (Parr, 2018). When you are overextended and overloading your schedule, it is difficult to even consider packing healthy snacks or lunches. Meal planning is a way to organize your weekly lunches in advance and to ensure healthy choices. These are strategies teachers can use to ensure they have nutritional boost midday.

- Plan and pack your lunches for the week on Sunday. That way, your daily task of preparing lunch is done in one chunk of time.
- When making dinner for a family of four, prepare enough for six. That way, you'll have leftovers that you can easily warm up for lunch at school.
- Use the school refrigerator. If you don't mind eating the same thing all week, bring a batch of soup and keep it in the refrigerator. Nobody said food stored in the teachers' lounge has to be in individual portions.

Use the Gym Equipment

Many schools have physical education supplies such as jump ropes, hand weights, basketballs, and yoga mats. Some schools even have weight rooms with equipment. Take advantage of the resources that your school has available and spend some time using the equipment. This is a quick way to add more activity into your routine without the increased time and cost of joining a gym.

Take It Outside

As we mentioned, sunshine is good for your physical health. The light increases alertness and fresh air cleans your lungs, reinforces your immune system, and can help clear your head (Smith, 2019). Look for opportunities to take your lesson outside.

If students have a lengthy piece of text to read or you are planning to use a lot of space or movement, determine if you can accomplish your lesson goals in the school's courtyard. Review your curriculum units for ways you can incorporate real-world methods and get active. For example, instead of growing plants in your classroom window, find a safe location outside and plant a garden. It doesn't matter if the plants are in the ground or they stay potted. The point is to have a reason to take advantage of the physical benefits gardening provides.

Another way to soak up the benefits of the great outdoors is to model the pride you have in your school and incorporate movement by dedicating the last 5–10 minutes of a lesson to picking up trash or other beautification efforts for your school grounds. When you have a day heavy with sitting, you and your students will benefit from the physical movement of walking and stretching needed to execute this small service project.

Don't Be Seated

An article published by the Better Health Channel (2018) was titled, "The Dangers of Sitting: Why Sitting is the New Smoking." The article states physical inactivity contributes to over three million preventable deaths each year and is the fourth leading cause of death due to non-communicable diseases.

If that isn't enough to get your attention, consider the statement from Cable News Network (CNN), Health that says, "No matter how much you exercise, sitting for excessively long periods of time is a risk factor for early death." It goes on to say, "There's a direct relationship . . . as your total sitting time increases, so does your risk of an early death" (Scutti, 2017).

Getting off your bum is not only about getting more movement. To be very clear with the research we found: Even if you are reasonably active, hours of sitting are harmful to your health. One study reported that one hour of intense exercise did not make up for the negative effects of inactivity when the other hours were spent sitting (Duvivier et al., 2013).

You might be wondering why the concept of sitting is mentioned to an audience of teachers in this book. Most teachers' days are spent standing and moving around in a classroom. Who has time to sit when we are educating the future? It's not the time during the school day that poses the most worry for teachers. It's after the bell.

The suggestion is not that you shouldn't take a load off and rest your feet after a long day of standing on them. What we do want you to think about is time spent grading papers, writing lesson plans, and reading and then responding to emails.

Duties that teachers have beyond instruction often are performed at a table or desk. And, these duties often require hours of time to complete. Given the research, it makes sense to take action to avoid the negative impact prolonged sitting produces. Here are some tips to keep in mind when you pull up a chair.

- When watching TV, stand or, if you choose to sit, try a stability ball
- During phone calls, use your speaker and make a point to stand up, even stroll when you're talking
- Set a timer to limit your sitting to no more than 30 consecutive minutes before you get up and stretch or move
- Use a standing desk or counter height table when you can
- Walk and talk when meeting with students or colleagues instead of using the conference room
- Break up tasks like laundry, dishes, or picking up the house rather than doing them all at once. They can be used to interrupt time that you might be seated too long
- Stand on the perimeter of the room rather than sit for long meetings

Drink Up

Your body is constantly losing water and you need to replenish. Approximately 60 percent of your body weight is made of water. A study by French and American researchers found that many adults are not drinking enough water (Heid, 2013). The amount of water you need varies for each person, but the Institute of Medicine recommends for men, 13 cups of fluid each day and for women, 9 cups of fluid each day (Marcin, 2019).

If you're having trouble drinking that much water, focus on just increasing your intake by one cup at a time. Some teacher tricks for consuming more water include having a water container handy as you're teaching and looking for opportunities to hit the water bottle.

- Pick a time during your lesson when you're having a class discussion. Every time a student speaks, take a sip.
- Carry your water bottle with you whenever you leave the classroom. You can't drink from it if it's left on your desk.
- Between lessons or classes, consume a half cup of water. Keep your water in a container that tracks capacity; this way you will be able to gauge how much you drink during the day.
- Place a water bottle in your car so it's readily available on your commute. Make a conscious effort to have water constantly accessible to you and make water your preferred drink choice.

Take a Bathroom Break

This might approach the limits of what you might expect in a book for teachers to discuss. But, it isn't good for you to hold it. We already mentioned that teachers, as a profession, get more urinary tract infections than other professions. Other consequences of ignoring your urge to pee include incontinence and urinary retention, which is when your bladder muscles are so tense they can't relax when you want them to.

Healthline states that emptying your bladder six to seven times a day is normal (Lou & Watson, 2019). Depending on the amount of fluid intake, your bladder could fill even more quickly. Monica Nelson (2013), health and fitness expert, shares this tip for the amount of water intake: take your body weight, divide it in half and drink that number in ounces of water. An adult bladder is considered full with 16–24 ounces, so you do the math on the number of bathroom breaks needed in a day.

Park from a Distance

Instead of trying to get the closest parking space to the school entrance, park in the last row of the parking lot. This will give you added movement and extra steps in your day. As you walk, take some deep breaths and focus on nature for a moment before entering the school building.

Prepare for a Snack Attack

Do you have a snack box or treat basket? How many times do you dip into it for a quick sugar fix or to try to quiet your hunger grumblings? Instead of raiding your snack cupboard for students, reserve a space for your own teacher snack drawer that has healthy snacks readily available for you.

No Homework

You read that right! Homework for them means homework for you. Reducing or eliminating homework for a night (or forever) will lessen your workload, giving you more time outside the school day to tend to your physical needs and other areas of wellness. As Sackstein and Hamilton (2016) point out, nightly homework also detracts from clubs, sports, and other activities that support students' physical activity as well. So, distract yourself from your homework and focus on self-care for you—the teacher.

Take a Recess Break

Joining your students outside during their recess has multiple benefits. First, it's a wonderful opportunity for you to see your students in a social environment and build relationships. But, in terms of self-care, going outside offers another way to get some physical activity packed into your day. When you make this play part of your routine, it strengthens your heart and reduces your stress.

Wash Your Hands

School buildings, even with the best custodial staff, are filled with germs. Teachers are exposed to environmental hotspots for germs and students that carry them. According to the CDC, school-aged children contract eight to twelve cases of cold or flu per year. That means every time they touch their face, or cough without covering their mouths, germs are scattered everywhere, just waiting to get you sick too.

As we learned in 2020 with the COVID-19 pandemic, frequent hand washing helps the prevention of viruses of any kind. If you don't have a sink in your classroom, a pump of hand sanitizer will do the trick. Consider establishing some classroom routines that help reduce the spread of germs. As you greet students at the door, encourage them to wash their hands before going to their desks, or welcome them with a dose of hand sanitizer.

Don't Stand and Deliver

You can get a twofer when you intentionally plan movement into your lessons. Students will benefit from gallery walks, silent discussion boards, and rotating stations, but they also afford you the chance to help blood flow and provide oxygen to the brain through movement too. If your classroom permits, set up more than one teaching area. Instead of having your whiteboard and your workstation close to one another, force yourself to walk back and forth from the computer to SmartBoard to help keep you moving.

TEAM UP FOR PHYSICAL CARE

If you're feeling on top of your game when it comes to physical wellness, you can take that energy and apply it to other areas of your personal well-being. Or, you might choose to leverage your benefit to support others who might welcome your guidance or encouragement.

Teaming up for physical care means you are choosing to help others to take the first steps or create opportunities for them to benefit from a good night's sleep, a nutritious meal, or some exercise. Their physical well-being is not your responsibility, but if this is an area where you thrive, sharing with others might give you a spiritual boost, which is explored more in chapter 5.

Read through this initial brainstorm of ways you might support your friends, family, or coworkers and team up for physical care.

Divvy Up Lunch Duty

Meal planning is associated with a healthier diet (Ducrot et al., 2017). Start a lunch club with a handful of colleagues. Assign each person a day of the week to provide a healthy lunch for everyone. Keep it low-key and simple. This isn't a strategy that should require hours of research and preparation. An example might be five turkey sandwiches, a bag of carrots, and a giant tub of yogurt with a side of granola to share. It's not about having a gourmet lunch, it's teaming together to help one another tend to your physical well-being.

Share Your Slumber Secrets

An online channel is a great way to connect with others with similar interests. There's a group for everything! If you have great ideas for falling asleep fast or are looking to narrow down the many apps to track the quality of your sleep, an online interest group might be just the place.

Host a Meal Swap

A meal swap is just like a cookie exchange, but with dinners! Instead of buying different ingredients for five meals, invite four friends or family members to each prep one healthy dish. Each meal is assembled and ready to cook, sometimes frozen. Host a swap party for everyone to come and trade meals. You will prepare five (or whatever number you chose) batches of vegetable soup, but by the end of the night, your fridge or freezer will be filled with five different meals ready for you to toss in the oven or crockpot. Do an Internet search for meal swap recipes to get great ideas for menu items that work best.

Sign Us Up

If you want to help others get more physical activity in their lives, a suggestion to show up at a local gym might be intimidating to anyone who doesn't know how to use the equipment. You might have more luck inviting them to take a class. See if your community education offers classes that combine exercise and fun. Consider a dance, yoga, or fitness class. Local gyms often offer beginner classes too. If you agree to go with them, they are more likely to go and you just might find that you love kickboxing or whatever you decide to try.

Night on the Town

Instead of going to dinner and a movie, choose activities with your partner that include movement. Picnic lunch (packed or takeout) followed by a stroll through the park. Use your imagination, the sky's the limit, and even skydiving is an option; roller skating, rock climbing, dancing, laser tag, or a trip to a trampoline park are other choices.

Put Your Potluck on a Diet

Potluck lunch in the teachers' lounge isn't exactly known for its health benefits. We often see a table of desserts and another table for everything else. To encourage others to enjoy lunch without overloading on calories, announce a potluck dedicated to showcasing food on the healthier side. Then, start a Google Doc and invite your coworkers to upload the recipes for the dish they brought. Now everyone has a collection of menu items they have tried, enjoyed, and can make again at home or for another gathering.

Take It Inside

Connie and Dorothy both live in Michigan where there are four distinct seasons. They find it easy to correlate activities to different times of the year. It's common to water ski in the summer and sled in the winter. Consider the weather where you live. Keep your family active while planning something unexpected. If it's hot, look for an indoor ice rink and go skating. If it's snowing outside, plan a trip to an indoor pool. Don't let the forecast restrict you from your favorite outdoor activities.

Naptime Nanny

Do you have a friend, colleague, or loved one who is feeling under the weather? They might appreciate an offer for their kids to have a sleepover at your place. Giving someone peace and quiet in their own home to catch up on some needed zzzs could make a big difference in nursing themselves back to good health. If the night hours are not the problem, consider a play date with the kids instead, so your sick friend can relax or take a daytime nap.

Deliver It Hot and Ready

Tragedy can strike at any time. When a loved one is hospitalized, the stress of working, managing a family, and spending time in the hospital takes a toll on a person's sleep schedule. And, let's face it, hospital food has improved, but it's not exactly a home-cooked meal. If a neighbor or someone you know is facing a situation you know is draining them, the gesture to provide a home-cooked meal can be more impactful than you know.

One meal you give saves them time, fuels their body with nourishment, and will let them feel cared for as they are caring for someone else. You can either provide a meal that can be eaten out of the refrigerator or easily heated up, or meet them at the door when they get home with the hot meal ready to serve. Disposable containers work best. No dishes and no obligation to return them. Remember—part of your gift is time, so this is not the opportunity to get the scoop on how their loved one is doing. Drop off the food and leave quickly, unless they directly invite you to stay because they need the companionship themselves.

FEATURE THE TEACHER WITH PHYSICAL WELLNESS

Three sixth grade teachers in Saranac Community Schools detested packing their lunch every day. Saranac, Michigan, is a town of 1409 people, which is not enough to support even one drive-thru restaurant. If you don't bring your lunch, your choices are to buy a school lunch or go hungry.

In a 30-minute duty-free lunch, who wants to spend five of them waiting for an available microwave and another eight preparing your unappetizing frozen meal? Scarfing down sweet and sour chicken from a plastic container in less than ten minutes and still leave time to check your mailbox, go to the bathroom, and get back to your classroom before lunch is over doesn't make for a relaxing break from the strains of teaching.

So Sue Chipman, Amy McGee, and Carol Webb started a salad club. Instead of individually packing their lunches, they each signed up to bring a few salad ingredients every Monday. One person would bring leafy greens and cheese, someone else would bring veggies, and a third would bring a protein such as boiled eggs or grilled chicken. They changed it up slightly each week, adding toppings like quinoa, sunflower seeds, or nuts.

The teachers kept their items in the refrigerator all week. Then, every day at lunch, one of them would pull out the ingredients, set them on the lunch table, and salads would be made! Anyone who wanted to join the salad club could be a member simply by contributing to the salad buffet on Monday. What started with just the three teachers quickly became a lunch break salad party that included administration and support staff.

Minimal prep, healthy lunch, and comradery during lunchtime had a positive trickle-down effect. The salad club members had more time with their families in the evening that used to be spent deciding what to pack for lunch, then actually packing it. They were also fueled by the salad's nutrients to maintain the stamina to teach sixth grade. Perhaps the biggest benefit of all was the teachers were able to enjoy each other's company during their afternoon meal.

EDUCATOR COMMITMENT TO PHYSICAL WELL-BEING

At the beginning of the chapter, questions were provided to help you process what you are reading. Now, use these questions to reflect on what you learned and what connections you are making to your personal physical self-care and wellness.

1. How has my definition of physical wellness been confirmed or shifted?
2. What are some ways I can intentionally build my physical well-being?

3. What a-has did I have about sleep, diet, or movement?
4. What are the most doable steps I can take to improve my physical health?

To provide additional reflection, the Physical Care Needs Assessment Checklist in Table 1.2 asks you to pause and record the frequency in which you experience the listed statements. The checklist will reveal where you have developed habits (both healthy and unhealthy), where you are developing habits, and areas where more care for your physical well-being might be necessary. You might want to revisit this chart as events in your life occur or you make changes to your routine.

Table 1.2: Physical Care Needs Assessment Checklist

	Never/ Rarely	Occasionally	Frequently/ Always
I maintain a balanced diet.			
I drink enough water each day.			
I resist unhealthy snack choices.			
My overall health is monitored by my doctor.			
I have a bedtime and morning routine.			
I am often tired.			
I have difficulty falling asleep.			
When I wake up, I feel refreshed.			
My muscles are limber and flexible.			
I am strong.			
I am easily winded.			
I take any medicine I am prescribed as directed.			
I have an exercise routine.			
I don't sit for more than 30 consecutive minutes.			
Exposure to blue light is limited in the evening.			
I plan meals in advance.			
There is a specific place I go to exercise.			
I eat two–three cups of vegetables daily.			
I have strong willpower.			
I fit in 150 minutes of moderate exercise every week.			
I eat on a schedule.			
I have exposure to sunshine daily.			
I take measures to prevent getting sick.			
When I nap, I still feel groggy.			
I intentionally tend to my physical wellness.			
I can recognize when I need a physical boost.			
My physical care backpack has strategies that help me in this area of wellness.			

In future chapters, the benefits and formats of journals will be shared. The journaling activity described in this chapter provides you a picture of what's happening around you and how that might impact your ability to focus on your physical care. In a notebook, create three columns. Record the date in the first column. Over time, you will be able to identify patterns of events that impact you and in what ways.

The second column is for reflection. In the Reflection column, think about where you are today and how that has influenced your sleep, diet, exercise, or medical health. Be sure your entry is free of judgement. For example, in mid-August, you might be reflecting on how a summer schedule influences your physical wellness. You might write:

> *August 15: Over the summer I had more flexibility over my schedule. When I worked in the garden, I exercised and felt like I was productive. The freedom to eat whenever I want has made my diet less healthy than it should be. I get so excited about the new school year that sometimes I can't sleep at night.*

To prepare for goal-setting, the final column in your journal entry brings your attention to your immediate future. Think specifically about changes you can anticipate that might cause a shift in the way you tend to your physical wellness. You will use the information in this journal entry to develop goals and commit to yourself and your physical well-being.

> *As I get ready for back-to-school, I will be able to get on a better eating schedule, but fitting in exercise is always a struggle. I have to make sure I get at least seven hours of sleep every night.*

Review your needs assessment checklist and your three-column journal entries. Think about each area of self-care individually. Based on this reflection, choose where you are on the Physical Meter Assessment Levels in Figure 1.5. Your physical care is broken into four categories that contribute to your overall physical health: sleep, diet, movement, and medical. There is not a right or wrong answer so place yourself in the area that makes the most sense for you.

In the categories where you have a need to improve, prioritize your most important areas. Do you need to change your patterns? If so, return to the portion of the chapter where we offer ways to build habits. In this chapter, the heading is "Getting Into a Physical Groove." If your needs feel more temporary and a short-term fix is a better approach, you'll find those tips in the "When You Need a Physical Surge" section.

Use the suggestions offered to select how you will give attention to yourself in the area of physical self-care. Take the ideas as they are or tweak them to

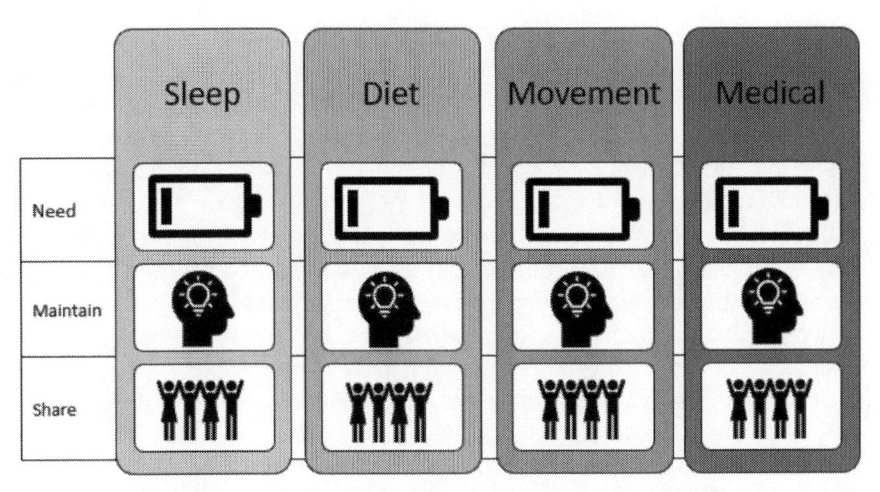

Figure 1.5: Physical Meter Assessment Levels. *Source:* Connie Hamilton

fit your style and circumstances. If you read something that inspires a different idea for you, great. There isn't a one-size-fits-all, so any personalization you make will increase the likelihood that the custom plan will work for you.

There may be some areas where you're feeling pretty confident. No problems, but maybe you're not excelling yet. In this case, you will likely select "maintain" as your assessment level. Your focus in the areas in the *maintain* category is exactly as it sounds. Keep up the good work without neglecting areas of your physical well-being to tend to others. For example, maybe you're consistently getting seven or eight solid hours of sleep at night.

Perhaps another area needs attention, like movement. If you decide to hit the gym before school each day, the alarm going off at 5 am could cut into a good night's sleep. Prevent the robbing Peter to pay Paul phenomenon by mindfully maintaining the areas where your physical well-being is meeting your goals. To accomplish this, protect contributors to your success. Keep those strategies in your metaphorical physical wellness backpack.

As you began this chapter, you probably had a hunch of what areas of your physical wellness are solid. Maybe even exceptional. In the circumstances when you have found your groove and are excited about it or are very passionate about a specific area of your personal well-being, we encourage you to consider the option to share that passion with others.

It is unlikely you will land in the "share" category for every area of self-care. If you did, you probably wouldn't have chosen to read this book. However, it is helpful to recognize the multi-layered benefits that sharing with others can provide such as a sense of contributing to the greater good. If there is an area within your physical well-being that warrants a "share" label, "Team Up for Physical Care" offers a menu of ways you can pay it forward.

A physical self-care plan is not going to be set in stone. Your needs will fluctuate. The short and long-term effects of the care (or lack of care) you give to yourself will be noticed. It only takes one night of no sleep to find yourself in need of some physical TLC. Some other areas might take longer to surface. A consistently poor diet isn't going to show up on your bathroom scale in one morning.

Instead, the slow impact will creep up and has the potential to go unnoticed. Preparing a plan to ensure you pay attention to your physical well-being is one way to avoid unwanted results of inattention to your body's needs.

People who set goals are more likely to achieve them (Matthews, 2015). Hence, some tools have been provided to help you select your goals to improve your physical well-being. As you use the tools, develop a picture of how to champion your physical health. It's time to make a commitment to yourself. Specifically, your physical wellness.

Chapter 2

Attention on Emotional Health

Do emotions impact your actions or do actions impact your emotions? To be honest, this is a little bit of a chicken-and-egg scenario because the answer is not straightforward. Emotions are very scientific. Chemical, to be more specific. How you feel is largely determined by what the chemicals in your brain are doing. Your brain often responds without you thinking about it. These automatic actions by your brain are called unconscious processes. Although you do not have complete control over your emotions, the good news is, they can be managed. Awareness of your emotions is the first step in determining how to change or cope with them.

Emotional self-care includes engaging in activities that help you connect, process, and reflect on a range of emotions. When emotions are flaring high, there is a tendency to become impulsive. Many people understand that it is important to have a good diet, exercise, and rest, but often overlook emotional wellness. This chapter will circle back around to the introduction and the emotional reasons teachers chose to enter the field.

The excitement of a career in education can dwindle quickly without tending to your own needs. Paying attention to emotional wellness for teachers is essential. One out of four teachers indicated they considered leaving teaching after the 2020–2021 school year (Hess, 2021), but the pandemic is not solely to blame. Prior to the pandemic, approximately one out of six teachers in America were likely to leave the profession. It is time to view self-care as a necessity, not a luxury.

Teachers need self-care strategies to thrive and avoid feeling strained and drained. This chapter will include ideas for teachers to incorporate emotional wellness and self-care into their routines. As you progress throughout the chapter you will once again see guiding questions to enhance your learning experience. The guiding questions for this chapter help evoke what you already understand about emotional wellness. Your thoughts will help highlight what your experiences and knowledge bring to the conversation about emotional wellness while opening opportunities for you to add to your understanding or look at emotional care in a new way.

1. What is my current definition of emotional wellness?
2. How do I tend to my emotional well-being?
3. What perception do I have of emotional health?
4. What is something I hope to learn as I read?
5. How would I rate my current emotional well-being barometer?

YOUR STATE OF MIND

In order to understand why the strategies outlined in this chapter are helpful, you will need to grasp how the brain works in terms of your emotions. Your beautiful brain acquires information from your senses and your emotions. Your senses help make you aware of what is happening in the world, your emotions guide you to determine what these circumstances mean to you. Emotions drive you to take care of needs such as safety and companionship.

Endorphins are your body's natural pain reliever; they are molecules associated with pain relief produced by pituitary and hypothalamus glands in your brain. Endorphins prompt positive feelings in the body and are released when you do something you enjoy. Oxytocin is a hormone produced by the brain and associated with maternal behavior and social behavior. These brain chemicals help us feel good. Emotional care goes beyond the idea of happiness. Emotions create an awareness of what needs attention and emotional self-care encompasses acknowledging all of these feelings, which include those that feel joyful and some that are painful.

Your emotions help you identify danger, influence decisions, and understand other people. When you feel frightened, depressed, angry, anxious, or tense, your body's response is to release stress hormones. The hormones include adrenaline and cortisol, which prepare your body to cope with the stress you are feeling. You may find your heart beats faster and your blood vessels narrow to push blood to the center of the body. The flight-or-flight response you feel is assumed to date back to prehistoric times when humans needed to escape predators. Clearly, we do not want to live in a constant state of hyper-awareness and fear. However, these emotions are needed to help people identify danger quickly, then deescalate when it's safe.

It is critical to have the skills to reflect on and regulate your emotions. You want to have healthy ways to express your feelings. You don't want to stifle feelings. Suppressing your emotions makes you aggressive and easily agitated (University of Texas, 2011, Raypole, 2020). For example, if you squelch feelings of frustration toward your principal at school, you are more likely to be snippy or start an argument with your partner at home.

In an attempt to block this feeling, the emotion is actually building up inside of you, which may lead to feeling the emotion unexpectedly later on. This sequence of events makes many people feel like they are not in control. Emotional self-care can help you regulate daily stress and mental health challenges such as anxiety or depression (Gobin, 2019). Your conscious self can impact how your brain understands how to identify reactions to negative emotions, then mindfully and intentionally trigger actions that solicit more positive emotions. It is important to care for your emotional needs by identifying what you are feeling and how to best address these feelings.

Physical responses to negative emotions like fear, frustration, and disgust such as sweating, increased heart rate, and rapid breathing tell you that something is wrong. It is your body's way of sending you a message and protecting you. Emotions exist for a reason; your body is taking care of you in a similar way when you feel emotional pain. Lysa Terkeurst (2018), author of *It's Not Supposed to Be This Way*, writes:

> The feeling of the pain is like a warning light on the dashboard of our car. The light comes on to indicate something is wrong. We can assume it's a little glitch in the operating panel. We can even go to the mechanic and ask him to turn off that annoying little light. But if he's a good mechanic, he would tell you it's foolish not to pay attention to it. Because if you don't attend to it, you will soon experience a breakdown. The warning light isn't trying to annoy you. It's trying to protect you. (p. 36)

Do not dismiss feelings—listen to what your emotions are trying to tell you. Then determine what the feelings mean, how they are impacting your overall well-being, and how you should respond to them.

FLOODING YOUR LIFE WITH EMOTIONAL CARE

When people wait for their emotions to have a negative impact on their lives, they live in a reactionary state. Establishing habits and routines that flood your life with mindful ways to address your emotional needs provides you the opportunity to prevent emotions from draining you. Additionally, a positive and optimistic lifestyle helps build resilience and reduces the impact stress has on you.

A proactive approach strengthens your emotional ability to deal with curveballs and stressors that are inevitable in your role as an educator and your personal life. Nourish your inner self so you can flourish. Review these options for caring for your emotional well-being. Choose an example that seems easy to implement and begin to incorporate the strategy into your routine. Then, try another that might take a little more effort and see if you can create a new habit that nurtures your emotional care as you build your wellness backpack.

Self-Affirmations

Words matter. You must treat yourself as kindly as you treat your students, parents, or your favorite colleagues. Teachers support students in so many ways and are often the stable force in their lives. Teachers serve others constantly and are encouraging to students and staff. Yet, educators frequently overlook their own needs and keep moving forward meeting the needs of others.

Be kind and speak graciously to yourself. Give yourself a message of strength and hope. Try using self-affirmations. Self-affirmations are encouraging statements or phrases that are meant to guide you to positive thoughts. They make you less likely to dismiss harmful health messages, focusing instead to the intention to change for the better (Silverman et al., 2013; Harris and Epton, 2009).

Your affirmations could be written on sticky notes on your mirror, computer, or in a journal. Determine the best place for you to view and read the affirmations on a regular basis. In order to make lasting, long-term changes to the ways you think and feel, positive affirmations require regular practice (Moore, 2021). Sometimes you might get stuck on a detrimental comment from a colleague, friend, parent, or family member. Don't allow pessimistic attitudes of others' disheartening words to define your thinking. Because self-affirmations have been shown to decrease stress levels (Critcher & Dunning, 2015) and they don't take much time or effort, it's worth a try.

Sample Self-Affirmations

- I am capable of amazing things.
- My influence on students is endless, I choose to model kindness and hope.
- I can accomplish anything I set my mind to.
- I know I am a good teacher and I have a passion for children.
- I try to see the best in others.
- I decide how I feel and today I am choosing happiness.
- I can be strong and have the ability to connect with my most difficult students.
- I am confident I can help guide our principal in a positive direction.

Get a Professional

When you are overly stressed and frustrated, it is easy to vent to a colleague or someone close to you. These people are often there for you and truly care about you, but they may not be equipped to offer unbiased input. It is completely normal to talk to your support circle about what is on your mind, but if you are feeling your emotions are getting in the way of your happiness or daily life, a counselor or therapist is better equipped to help you develop productive coping skills. A mental health professional can help you hone in on areas of your emotional health that you want to improve and get you on the right path to developing a plan.

Tend to Your Other Areas of Self-Care

Each chapter in this book is dedicated to a different aspect of your overall well-being. However, these components, as mentioned in the introduction, are not mutually exclusive. Physical activity, as discussed in chapter 1, creates endorphins that provide a good feeling. Ever heard of a "runner's high"? Likewise, you will learn in chapter 4 how social interactions also impact emotions. So paying attention to the other areas of your personal wellness will help create emotional stability or an outlet to release negative emotions in a healthy way.

Grow Your Mindset

Paying attention to your mindset is an important component of self-care. Emotional mindsets show strong associations with mental health (DeFrance, 2020). A growth mindset, defined by Carol Dweck, is a belief that abilities and intelligence can be developed. This mindset is often portrayed in contrast with a fixed mindset, which is the belief that abilities and intelligence are predetermined at set intervals (Dweck, 2006).

Contrary to common misunderstanding, individuals aren't labeled as having a growth mindset or a fixed mindset. We don't walk around in a growth mindset. When faced with a challenge, how the challenge is perceived, then the actions taken to address the challenge, are good indications of what type of mindset is being applied. Recognizing when fixed thoughts inhibit you is one way to build a habit of growth-minded thinking. Likewise, as obvious as it might sound, a growth mindset can't empower you to leap tall buildings with a single bound. Therefore, not every challenge can be overcome with mindset alone.

You might recognize these words from the Serenity Prayer. It also supports one of four ways that dialectical behavior therapy (DBT) therapists teach their clients to approach problems. When faced with an issue about anything, from being overwhelmed to feelings of isolation or dealing with an undesirable situation, DBT suggests you have four options:

1. *Solve the Problem*: This might include changing a situation, figuring out a resolution, or simply removing yourself from the situation altogether. For example, if you aren't able to greet students as they enter the class and distribute laptops to them at the same time, you might solve the problem by assigning a student to distribute laptops so you aren't trying to accomplish two things at once.
2. *Feel Better About the Problem:* You can decide to leave the situation as it is, but mindfully change how you think about it. For example, if you're asked to teach a class you've never taught before and are feeling overwhelmed with the idea of writing the curriculum from scratch, you might shift your perspective to look at the opportunity as an honor to be asked and embrace the chance to connect with students through different content.
3. *Tolerate the Problem:* Here is where the ability to accept things you cannot change comes in. Sometimes problems will be out of your control to solve and you might not be able to flip your emotions from dislike to elation. However, you can choose to accept reality and avoid emotional suffering. For example, when the master schedule is completed, you might detest the sequence of classes or where your planning period is within the day. Tolerating the problem allows you to accept the schedule the way it is and move on. You don't have to like it, but perseverating on it is a choice you make to feed your own negative emotions.
4. *Stay Miserable:* While this is not a good option, it is an option. Not only can you choose to stay miserable, but in many cases, the way people respond causes their problems to get worse. For example, if you are faced with a short deadline for a complex task and you choose to spend an hour venting to a colleague about how you don't have enough time to get the project done, you have even less time to get the job done, making the problem worse than it was an hour ago.

Using these DBT problem-solving options as a way to approach difficulties on a regular basis helps you develop mindfulness about the choices you make to deal with a problem. If you recognize that you are unable to let go of something that has you riled up, ask yourself how you want to address the problem. Just being aware of how you are coping (or not coping in the case of staying miserable) can move you to a healthier state of mind.

Know the Social Media Perspective

The effects of social media are concerning. Research finds that there is a direct correlation between depression and increased use of social media, especially for those who are predisposed to depression (Hartanto et al., 2021). Oftentimes we see the staged version on social media and not the reality of what is happening behind the scenes. This artificial positivity causes viewers to compare their lives to the edited, filtered, and carefully worded posts they read.

Exposure to touched up selfies and photos that give the appearance of storybook lives sparks comparison. People's natural lives don't typically reflect the spruced-up versions they post. However, that doesn't prevent followers from comparing their natural lives to the spruced-up versions they see and read about others. The apples-to-oranges crosswalk leads many to a feeling of inadequacy.

If you find yourself imagining how wonderful someone's life must be based on their social media posts, remember they get to choose what they post. The selection process for what makes it to an Instagram post likely involves meeting a very high criteria. Ask yourself to estimate how many photos or daily events were passed up because they exposed imperfections in someone's life. That might give you the perspective needed to discourage you from comparing yourself to their post.

Chart Your Mood

Keeping track of how you're feeling from day to day can reveal patterns in events that lift you up or bring you down. There is a sample at the end of this chapter, or you can do an Internet search for "mood tracker" and find a format to your liking. In your first week, notice if your mood is constant or fluctuates in the morning or evening. After your first month of logging, look to see if any patterns emerge on certain days of the week.

The data you gather through this activity will empower you to better prepare for days or times of day when you are more likely to need an emotional boost. A proactive approach to coping keeps you in control. Your preparedness also reduces the potential for a situation to catch you off guard and trigger unhealthy stress levels.

Label Emotions

Make it your practice to accurately label your emotions. In 2000, Hariri conducted a study where participants were shown various facial expressions. One group was asked to match a picture of a face similar to the face they were shown. The other group identified linguistic labels instead of pictures, naming the emotion. The study was intended to look at the difference between instinctive emotional reactions when engaged in a perceptual task (matching pictures) versus an intellectual task (assigning a word that describes the expression).

When shown pictures of angry or frightened expressions, the first group showed an increase in regional cerebral blood flow (rCBF) in the amygdala, which is the brain's primary fear center. The other group, who named the expression, showed a diminished rCBFin the amygdala. It then triggered an increase in rCBF in the right prefrontal cortex. This is where emotions are regulated.

The results of this study suggest that naming expressions initiates the process of emotional regulation. Studies completed after Hariri validated the results and concluded that simply labeling an effect decreased negative emotions felt (Lieberman et al., 2011) and reduced physical reactions such as increased heart rate, rapid breathing, or perspiration that often accompanies negative emotions (Constantinou et al., 2014).

When labeling how you feel, try to be as specific as possible. An emotion wheel, provided by the Junto Institute, is shown in Figure 2.1. The inner ring shows categories of emotions. Then, as the wheel extends, the labels for the emotions get more specific. The cognitive effort to find the best word that describes your emotion will engage you intellectually. Are you really feeling scared or would a better descriptor be excluded, insignificant, or exposed?

WHEN YOU NEED AN EMOTIONAL DEPOSIT

Coping skills are what help you to regulate your emotions. There is not a one-size-fits-all formula for preventing your emotions from causing you to feel overly strained. However, if there were a formula, it would undoubtedly include recognizing the need to activate a coping strategy. Signs that your emotions are draining you might surface cognitively. High levels of stress and overwhelming emotions can make it difficult to concentrate or clearly identify a problem. There will be more on cognitive wellness in the next chapter. As mentioned in chapter 1, sustained levels of stress can lead to lack of sleep, increased or decreased appetite, and a general feeling of fatigue.

When other areas of your self-care are not tended to, you can experience more intense emotions or your emotions might be more easily triggered. Sometimes other areas of your health surface as emotional needs. In times when you need a boost in your emotional well-being, the strategies offered here might give you a temporary emotional deposit in your declining mood bank.

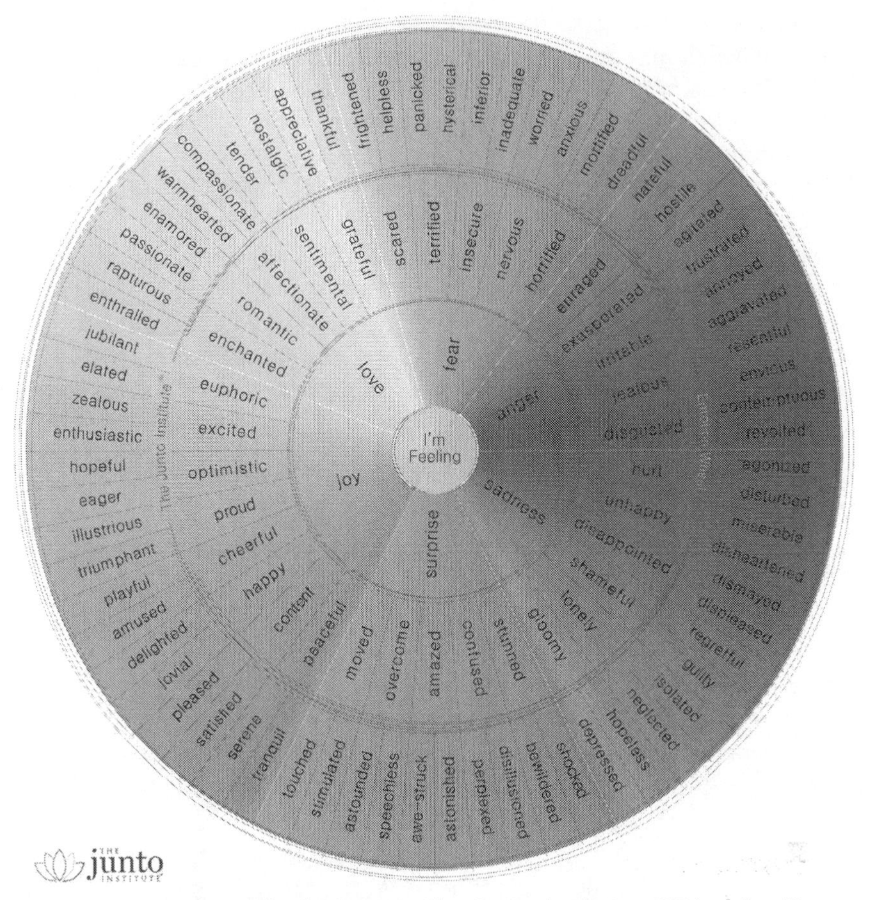

Figure 2.1: Emotion Wheel. ***Source:*** **The Junto Institute, 2021. https://www.thejuntoinstitute.com/emotion-wheels/**

Call a Helpline

If you are having thoughts of hurting yourself or others, don't wait for your next therapy appointment. Reach out to a helpline and get the support you need in the moment. The National Suicide Prevention Lifeline is open 24/7 and can be reached at 1-800-273-8255.

Check the Mirror

How you feel is likely written all over your face. Being strained can cause you to walk around with a scowl or generally unhappy face. The phenomenon of individuals mimicking the nonverbals of someone else is called mirroring and is often subconscious. You might exude sour energy without realizing it.

Maybe you're thinking about something causing you stress when walking down the hall. Your face will form an expression based on your thoughts, and your stride can portray the tension you're feeling. This, in turn, can trigger others to mirror your emotions creating a general sense of negativity.

Fortunately, the opposite is also true. When someone is animated and lively, those around them tend to align their actions to equal the level of energy shared. The same is true for gestures, speech patterns, and attitudes. When we ask someone why they're laughing, we often do it with a smile or a giggle. We are mirroring their happiness, even without knowing the reason for it, because laughter is contagious. So be aware not only of the sentiment you're depositing into your environment, but more importantly for your emotional wellness, how others are fueling your mood simply by being around you.

Be Positively Grateful

Gratitude helps block toxic emotions, such as resentment, envy, regret, and depression (Emmonds, 2010). By expressing gratitude, teachers can boost their feelings of optimism and reduce anxiety. A habit of gratitude allows you the opportunity to feel more satisfied and accomplished, and less emotionally exhausted. Practicing gratitude invites joy into our own lives, which means not just saying "I have the attitude of gratitude," but doing tangible things to practice gratitude (Brown, 2010).

Start a Smile

Turn that frown upside down. Fake it until you make it. These are cliché and corny, but they do offer good advice. Research has demonstrated that the simple act of smiling can lower your stress, lift your mood, and boost your immune system (Spector, 2017). Smiling is a simple task to do and it has huge payoffs for your emotional health. That smile promotes a chemical reaction in the brain, releasing specific hormones including dopamine and serotonin.

Dr. Gupta, a neurologist from IGEA Brain and Spine, shares, "Dopamine increases our feelings of happiness. Serotonin release is associated with reduced stress. Low levels of serotonin are associated with depression and aggression. Low levels of dopamine are also associated with depression" (Spector, 2017). When you need that emotional boost in positivity, smiling, whether forced or genuine, generally works well.

Walk Away

If things are feeling too emotional in the moment, a temporary break will be better in the long run. Understanding your emotions and knowing when it is a good idea to walk away is a form of protecting yourself. This will give you an opportunity to step away and process the situation from a distance.

Reach Out to Someone You Trust

There are times when you get an emotional boost by talking to a trusted friend or colleague. It is a gift to have a close confidant in your life that you are able to share your ups and downs with and know that you are in a safe space. However, a friend may mirror your perspective and it might be more helpful to seek a professional if you need more support.

Plan an Event

Think of an activity that you enjoy and plan an outing around the idea. This focus will give you something positive to look forward to as you embark on planning out a day for you and others to enjoy. It could entail something like visiting a museum or a day canoeing on the river.

Squirrel!

Can't stop thinking about one of the students in your class? Stressed about an upcoming family event? Worried about a contentious meeting next week? With all the things going on in the lives of educators, it is understandable that many are looking for ways to shift their thoughts. It may be time to distract yourself to get your mind off what's bothering you. Worrying about something coming up is a common source of anxiety. A temporary reprieve from fretting over future events might just give you the reboot you need to address the stress more easily. These activities are likely to distract your strained brain:

- Take a nap
- Call or Facetime a loved one
- Play with a pet
- Go shopping
- Engage in physical activity
- Check off a task from your to-do list like yard work, meal prep, or cleaning
- Enjoy your hobby

- Get outside and hike, enjoy a sunset, or watch kids play
- Reorganize a closet or drawer
- Play a game
- Dance
- Walk

Reread a Book or Rewatch a Favorite Movie

Movies or sitcoms are a way to temporarily escape the feelings busy teachers often face. When you're needing an emotional boost, watch old episodes of *The Office* and give yourself a break from whatever is draining your energy. Here are some suggestions:

- Carve out 20 minutes before bed tonight to read or listen to your favorite parts of books you've read. When you're ready to turn it off and head to sleep, tee up another section you want to revisit so it's ready to go next time.
- Take a familiar book with you to your doctor, dentist, or hair appointment. While you're waiting for your appointment, review your annotations and remember what resonated with you the first time you read it.
- Turn on a movie that lifts your heart or a sitcom that always makes you chuckle. Sit and watch it or have it on in the background while you fold laundry or tend to other tasks.

Partake in Comforting Activities

Certain activities can be counted on to bring you peace, relaxation, or joy. These events or places are unique to each person. Think of an experience or location that puts you in a calming state of mind. Some educators have offered the following ideas:

- Take a bath
- Visit a special spot
- Prepare a favorite meal
- Connect with family or friends
- Float in a pool
- Snuggle under a blanket
- Sit by a campfire
- Stroll through a park

If you can't physically go to your happy place, imagery is a strategy that can also cool nerves or allow you to cope with heavy emotions.

Release Through Sweat, Ink, or Tears

Some days your head may feel like a pressure cooker, ready to explode. There are a variety of safe outlets that release pent-up energy. Individuals choose decompression activities that range from strenuous exercise to journaling, or just a good cry. Let's explore how each of these options achieves the same outcome of easing your emotional well-being.

Release Through Sweat

The previous chapter highlighted the physical benefits of an active lifestyle. Unfortunately, the results most of us hope to gain by increased exercise, like losing weight or improving stamina, might take months to see. However, the emotional boost that exercise provides is almost instant. Michael Otto, Ph.D., a professor of psychology at Boston University, says we reap the most reward for a workout when we are feeling down. He says, "Failing to exercise when you feel bad is like explicitly not taking an aspirin when your head hurts. That's the time you get the payoff" (Weir, 2011).

You may opt to do something physical such as swimming to release some of your emotions. Aerobic exercises such as kickboxing or jogging have been linked to positive feelings and improved mental health (Santos-Longhurst, 2019). As always with any exercise, begin slowly and consult with your doctor to see if they have any concerns.

Release Through Tears

Paying attention to your emotions and having a way to let off steam before you blow is in your best interest. One way to blow off some steam is to let the tears flow. It is okay to cry. In the United States, women cry an average of 3.5 times per month and men cry an average of 1.9 times per month (Burgess, 2017). A good cry can make you feel better. Research shows that crying activates the parasympathetic nervous system, which helps people relax (Gracanin, et al., 2014). Not only is crying self-soothing, but shedding emotional tears releases endorphins and oxytocin. So crying provides the natural flow of brain chemicals that improve your mood.

Release Through Ink

Another outlet that might be a helpful technique for you is to pause and journal. Studies have found that journaling can lead to better sleep, a stronger immune system, and more self-confidence (Phelan, 2018). By focusing on mindful moments in writing, teachers can learn to express themselves privately. As you develop a deeper awareness of your current state of thought, you cultivate a sense of calmness and purpose in your life. Journaling can help teachers calm the mind, provide a safe space for thoughts, explore ideas, and create an opportunity for reflection. Not only does journaling allow a daily account of your thoughts, feelings, and life, but you are able to express yourself by writing freely.

BELL-TO-BELL ATTENTION ON EMOTIONAL HEALTH

It can be challenging to feed your emotional health when you're at school. Sometimes school itself is the cause of your feelings of stress. Regulating your emotions and keeping yourself focused will require you to use coping skills when you're teaching, joining meetings, and preparing for students. Even when you have built habits to maintain your health when it comes to emotional care, you can not limit the care you give to yourself before and after school.

A variety of options exist for how you can prevent your emotions from draining you. Like their teachers, students also reap the benefits of a learning environment that is thoughtfully aware of how to prevent emotional strain and what to do if and when it surfaces during school. While this chapter is about you and tending to your emotional health, bringing strategies to your classroom that include students is a twofer—you and your students enjoy the opportunity to regroup and nurture this type of self-care. The following strategies are selected because they can easily be used in the midst of a busy school day.

Just Breathe

One sign that your nerves are impacting you is your breath. Short, shallow, and quick breaths from the chest increase when tensions rise. You can combat some of the physical signs of high emotions by simply breathing with purpose. When you're relaxed or sleeping, your breathing tends to be deeper, and your lungs are more expanded with every breath. This is called diaphragmatic or abdominal breathing. Abdominal breathing is not done through your chest; it involves—you guessed it—your abdomen. There are many breathing techniques that can lower an accelerated heart rate and help you keep your cool in times of heightened emotions.

Box Breathing

This is a deep breathing technique, also referred to as square breathing. Think of this as a four-step process for each breath. Exhale for four counts. Hold with empty lungs for four counts. Then, inhale slowly for four counts. Finally, hold your lungs full of air for four counts. Then repeat.

Lion's Breath

If you do yoga, you might be familiar with this type of breathing. When using lion's breath, you relieve tension and stress by stretching your entire face, including the jaw and tongue. Get in a kneeling position and sit back on the heels of your feet, bringing the palms of your hands to your knees, and sit tall. Inhale through your nose, and exhale strongly through the mouth and make a "ha" sound, stick out your tongue as far as possible towards your chin and lift your eyes upward toward your forehead. As with any poses, if uncomfortable, make it your own and use a variation of the technique.

Model Journaling

Many classroom teachers help their students set up journals. Writing journals, science journals, and creative journals are among the types of writing books students use. Consider how a private journal or communication journal might benefit your students. Personal journals might be used for students to plan and reflect on their school experiences. This type of writing is successful as a free flow or with a little guidance from a prompt or another source of inspiration. Because personal journals are private to the individual writing them, it's a perfect time for a teacher to jot down a few thoughts of her own.

Communication journals function as a written conversation between students and their teacher. The topic for written discussion can be open, or a specific response to a posted question. After students complete their entries, the teacher reads the journals and responds to the students. This ongoing journal communication is a way to build on the student-teacher relationship. The journal prompts may include questions, quotes, or scenarios for students to reflect on as they write.

Journaling facilitates personal growth and helps you build your empathy with others. The activity often cultivates a sense of calmness and serenity in the classroom. When strategically scheduled in the school day, some quiet lyric-free music can set the stage for focus and serve as a great transition from a high-energy activity to something quieter or calmer.

Let Your Apps Affirm

Many cell phones allow you to create folders to categorize your apps and icons. Instead of keeping the default folder names, personalize the categories with self-affirmations that make you smile or evoke positive emotions.

Some examples are: "I am strong"—this section can include your wellness apps. "I am connected"—the section could include your social media apps and anything that connects you to others. "I am money smart"—could be all your financial items. The sky's the limit; use your creativity in naming the categories that are pleasant for you.

Partner with a Mentor or Coach

Education is a team sport. Although it frequently feels very lonely. If you're getting down on yourself because of something that isn't going right with your instruction, seek out a peer to serve as a thought partner. You might have an assigned mentor or just someone whose teaching inspires you. Reach out to a colleague and see if you can pick his or her brain about a question you have or a problem you're trying to solve in your classroom. Be respectful of his time by asking to get his thoughts for about ten minutes or join you for a planning session during your prep time one day next week.

If you're lucky enough to have an instructional coach on staff, you have a built-in confidant. It's literally this person's role to partner with you. Reaching out for coaching doesn't mean you're weak or a bad teacher. Even the very best athletes benefit from their coaches' perspectives and experience. Sometimes the outside point of view is what makes the difference when identifying root causes and brainstorming solutions.

Speak Up

Life happens. Your cat got sick last night and you were not able to get the napkins you agreed to pick up for the staff luncheon. You had a huge fight with your partner and you did not grade the essays. You may have a school or personal situation that is causing your emotions to flare, and you can't focus. You are feeling overwhelmed. Asking for support is definitely okay to do. You don't have to share details of what's causing you to need some space in order to request it. It's as simple as, "I'm dealing with something personal so I'm going to request some extra grace today." There aren't many people who can't relate to having a hard time, and most people will be empathetic and will gladly extend extra care when you need it.

Take a Sick Day

This concept was suggested in chapter 1 if you are feeling physically sick, but being emotionally unwell may require a day away as well. The idea for taking time off is not to purposely deplete all your days with no intention. However, if you are feeling emotionally unable to work, staying home and focusing on yourself is probably a good option. If you're planning a mental health day, you will find it more productive if it is filled with positive experiences while reducing your stress. Years ago, it was often frowned upon to take a day off of work, but educators who focus on their own wellness understand it is important to have a healthy body and mind.

Get Lost in the Lesson

Teaching can provide a much-needed distraction from strains you might be feeling outside school. Allow yourself an emotional break by escaping the hustle and bustle of everyday life. They say time flies when you're having fun, so enjoy your students, your content, and the routine that a day in your classroom can offer.

SPREAD EMOTIONAL JOY

Everyone has areas of their personal wellness that come more naturally to foster than others. If your emotional health is an area of strength for you, exuding that puts you in the position to be a positive influence on others who might be drained emotionally. Your choice to intentionally spread joy and maintain a positive outlook bolsters your personal wellness too. This section focuses on ways you can encourage healthy emotional care for others, but the joy you experience through helping others is a bonus.

Perform Random Acts of Kindness

Take credit or anonymously plan to support someone emotionally specific or perfect strangers. Performing random acts of kindness has been shown to improve overall happiness and benefit our emotional well-being. Kindness has also been shown to also improve heart health and increase our longevity. Some ideas to get you started:

- Paint a rock with words of kindness and leave the rocks around your neighborhood or school.
- Write a thank you note and put it in a colleague's mailbox with a special treat.
- Cheer up a colleague with a special coffee or tea drink in the morning.
- Make cookies or dinner for someone.
- Prepare a small gift basket for a friend in need.
- Donate clothes you are not using to a shelter or family in need.
- Plan an event for someone who needs an emotional break.

Narrate Your Kind Thoughts

It seems simple, and it is. If it's in your nature to be more optimistic than others, here's your opportunity to shed light on an alternate view of a situation. Narrate your choice to be positive if you find yourself in a "downer" environment. You might normally choose to stay quiet in a heated conversation or offer a neutral comment like "That's one way to look at it." Spreading joy includes communicating opportunities to have a more positive outlook on scenarios. The alignment of your beliefs and your behavior provides peace and harmony within you. Chapter 5 talks more about spiritual well-being when your true self aligns with your actions.

Deliver Support or Gratitude

If you already live a grateful life, share your positive perspective. Doing so offers a double win for the receiver. Not only do they get the support they need or the gratitude they deserve, but you'll be modeling a behavior that helps foster a positive state of mind.

Check In on Others

Think about how you feel when someone texts or calls just to see how you are doing. They don't have an agenda; they are simply concerned about how you are feeling. You are likely tempted to provide a more authentic response than the standard "fine" when you know their inquiry comes from a place of care and concern. This simple gesture is a way to generate feelings in the receiver. When you check in on someone, it makes them feel valued, worthy, and appreciated. If you choose a phone call or video call, make sure you have time and that you are prepared to listen. Some suggestions to get the conversation started:

- What is circling around in your mind today?
- How are you feeling right now?
- What's something I can do for you during this hard time?
- Were you able to get in any exercise or movement this week?
- What happened today that made you feel happy?

Blog About It

Reading blogs that validate emotions a person might be coping with offers a sense of connection, hope, and inspiration. It is rarely true that someone is the only person who has experienced a certain situation or event that causes their emotions to go into overdrive. Feeling emotions, even negative ones, are part of what makes us human. It's when those emotions cause someone to make decisions in the moment that have harmful long-term implications or fail to consider logical thinking that is a concern.

Publicizing your life ventures might be exactly what someone needs to normalize their situation and build the courage to push through tough times or stressful events. Not everything that strains educators is negative. Some people might feel overwhelmed with planning all the fine details of a family vacation. If you have recently learned tips and tricks for the perfect getaway or can warn others of pitfalls as they plan their own trip, consider sharing a blog post to enable your readers to benefit from your experience.

Start a Book Club

Book clubs allow teachers to learn and connect with others. The benefits of book clubs can challenge your understanding and help you make new connections that you may have not contemplated before the book club discussion. Book clubs are another way to read, learn, and explore new texts. Whether you are participating in a book club or reading alone, there are many ways to incorporate reading into your routine. If you travel for conferences or if you have a long work commute, try listening to audiobooks or podcasts while on the road.

Spread Happiness

During the pandemic, the focus was on social distance and making sure you weren't spreading anything unhealthy. But, when it is safe to do so, connecting with others is beneficial for your state of joy. Scientist James Fowler and Harvard professor Nicholas Christakis found that happiness spreads between pairs of people and from a person to their friends, to their friends' friends, and then to their friends (Porath, 2016). Their research demonstrated that frequent superficial, face-to-face interactions can also powerfully influence happiness. There will be more on social wellness in chapter 4.

FEATURE THE TEACHER WITH EMOTIONAL WELLNESS

Before she could write words, Christine was doodling pictures everywhere. Scrap paper and backs of greeting cards served as a canvas for her "writing." The day she used the stairway wall for her doodles was the day her mother, whom she calls "Nana," introduced her to a special place that could hold all her doodling. Christine had her very first journal. It was a simple spiral-bound notebook, and it was the first of many journals she would fill over the years.

For nearly 45 years, Christine turned to her journals when she was moved to write. She didn't have a specific routine, but that didn't prevent her from juggling three or four journals at a time. Mrs. Christine Bemis was a second grade teacher in December of 2019 when her mother passed. For months, her grief separated her from the main outlet she had used throughout her life. She rarely journaled. Seven days a week she visited her mother's gravesite with notebooks and pens in hand. Winter in Massachusetts gets quite cold, but Christine would sit on a bench in the freezing weather just to be near her mother. Instead of words, tears poured onto the pages. She couldn't bring herself to write an entry.

In July the following year, Christine took a clean copy of Dorothy's book, *Permission to Pause,* to the cemetery. She had been facing some serious medical issues and her doctor encouraged her to focus on self-care. The guided journal provided a focus on positive things in her life and a way to work through her grief simultaneously. A focus on herself was needed and her journaling began to change. She used the journal to help her move forward. The outlet helped her through one of the most emotionally painful events of her life.

Now, years later, Christine still mourns the loss of Nana. She finds having a record of her emotional journey helpful. The past entries give her an appreciation of her growth and hold her accountable for maintaining self-care that contributes to her emotional and overall wellness. What started out as childhood doodling is now a habit that serves as a powerful coping skill for emotional strength.

EDUCATOR COMMITMENT TO EMOTIONAL HEALTH

Now that you're more familiar with ways to support your own emotional well-being, answer the following prompts to make your takeaways clear.

1. How has my definition of emotional wellness been confirmed or shifted?
2. What are some ways I can intentionally build my emotional well-being?
3. What new perspectives have I gained about emotional health?
4. What new learning have I acquired?

Now, apply your understanding of emotional wellness and reflect on your own self-care. Table 2.1 is designed to provide you with information and serve as a needs assessment.

Table 2.1: Emotional Care Needs Assessment Checklist

	Never/ Rarely	Occasionally	Frequently/ Always
I use self-affirmations.			
I have a safe method to manage stress.			
I see a professional for support.			
My emotional exhaustion interferes with my daily activities.			
I try to have a growth mindset when posed with a problem.			
I feel like I need an emotional break.			
I am in a toxic relationship.			
I often have an outburst I later regret.			
I express gratitude to others.			
I spend time with those I care about.			
I am open-minded and flexible.			
When I need a sick day, I take it.			
I allow myself to cry.			
I blog or write.			
I check in on others.			
I pamper myself when needed.			
I intentionally tend to my emotional wellness.			
I can recognize when I need an emotional boost.			
I have sufficient strategies to support my emotional care.			

Review your responses in Table 2.1. This is a snapshot of your emotional well-being. You can revisit this checklist as often as you'd like to help you see where you are strong and how you might choose strategies to prevent your emotions from draining you.

Emotion Tracker

Tracking your emotions has multiple benefits. First, it calls your attention to how you are feeling. This retrospect is the first step to mindfulness and brings an awareness of what emotions you are experiencing. Second, as mentioned previously in this chapter, labeling your emotions begins the regulation process for keeping your feelings from taking over. The goal is not to suppress emotions. It is healthy to feel genuine emotions and it is necessary to experience emotions, even negative ones, to help you work through difficult times. The concern comes when your emotions prohibit you from making good decisions or tending to your needs for long periods of time. The third benefit of charting your emotions is that it provides a visual image that can be studied to determine patterns in your emotions.

If you notice, for example, that you consistently feel confident on Wednesday nights, you can look more closely at the events that transpire that evening. Is Wednesday the day you attend a self-defense behavior class? Maybe it's something more subtle like Wednesday is the day you meet with your mentee and he soaks up your advice and experience helping you to feel the value you bring to a new teacher. The point is to connect the dots between what happens in your day and how it impacts your emotional wellness.

The opposite is also worth exploring. Perhaps, when you review a few months of emotion tracking, a trend appears. You might see a feeling of remorse at the beginning of the month. After careful thought, a link between this emotion and tending to your family's budget could make you wonder if seeing your credit card bill is bringing attention to the impact of your daily smoothie purchases.

The goal of this type of activity is not to rub salt in a wound, but to allow you the opportunity to determine if you want or need to make a change. It's very possible that when you weigh your options, you decide that the short-lived feelings of remorse can be quickly squashed by reminding yourself that a $7 daily investment starts your day off well and the vitamin boost you add to your order makes a difference in how you feel all day long.

Conversely, you might decide that the repentance you feel is something you want to avoid, so you might decide to start making your own smoothies at home so next month you won't feel guilty for your indulgences. Either decision wouldn't be possible without first identifying what the trigger was for the feeling of remorse in the first place.

There are a variety of templates for tracking your emotions in creative ways. A google search for "emotion tracker" will give you some options. The purpose of tracking emotions is more than just completing the template. The power lies in the analysis of the data you gather over time. Periodically look back and think about what might have caused certain emotions you logged.

Emotional Deposits and Withdrawals

Tending to your emotional self-care requires more than just identifying your feelings. Emotions are ever-changing, so develop a habit of recognizing how you're feeling and the impact it's having on you from day to day. Certain people, environments, activities, and circumstances can either support your emotional well-being or drain it. Take charge of choosing how you want to feel. Emotions are triggered by events.

It's perfectly normal to be moved to tears when you see a video clip of a United States Marine being reunited with his family. Likewise, people commonly feel a surge of panic if their computer holding all of their files suddenly won't boot up. Many events simply occur without your control.

However, there are ways people can create moments that are likely to produce feelings they desire or shift unwanted feelings to more favorable ones.

Deposits to your emotional care are things that boost your mood and bring you happiness. On a sheet of paper or dedicated journal page, make a list of specific emotions you enjoy experiencing. For example, you might include joy, amused, accepted, appreciated, or inspired. Next to each emotion, link as many events or activities that are likely to solicit that emotion. This journal entry can be used to sprinkle events into your schedule to provide you with ample opportunities to bring wanted emotions into your life.

Just as these positive emotions add to your emotional bank, other emotions drain it. Withdrawals can deplete you. The negative impact of certain circumstances can compound, especially when you are not intentionally contributing positive experiences to balance them. When you are exposed to events that are emotionally draining, you become impatient and can even feel mentally paralyzed. To offset inevitable withdrawals from your emotional care, plan to reframe scenarios.

The age-old assessment of your optimism or pessimism to see a glass as half full or half empty is surprisingly common in actual situations you might find yourself in. Try using the following sentence stem to flip your perspective from seeing the downside of things to noticing the upside. It might _____, but at least ______. Here are some examples you might relate to:

- It might take two hours to get my drivers' license renewed, but at least it only has to be done once every four years.
- It might have failed, but at least I know what to avoid next time.
- It might be a flight delay, but at least I am not driving 24 hours.

The strategy of combating a negative thought with a positive counter-thought takes what could have been a withdrawal from your mood bank and turns it into a deposit.

When you are in a situation that is bound to reduce your emotional bank, try to respond with something to redirect your thinking or your actions. If you know that listening to 80s classic rock gets you pumped up and ready to conquer the world, it makes sense to use that tactic to snap yourself out of a slump. Start a new journal entry, but this time identify actions you can take to distract negativity. Some other examples include sitting quietly in your favorite chair, calling a friend to talk it out, or getting your mind off it briefly by tending to a small task on your "to do" list like taking out the recycling or watering your plants. The idea is to purposefully shift your attention from the source of stress long enough to give yourself a fresh perspective.

People are not always fully aware of their emotions and how those emotions are impacting various areas of their lives. You might not notice that you're hypersensitive when you're being evaluated, or maybe you don't recognize that if you're running late, you tend to feel more frazzled than normal. The strategies shared in this chapter are to help you both identify when your emotional well-being needs care and be resilient when emotions bring you down.

Your emotions will fluctuate from day to day—even minute by minute. Being mindful of your emotions positions you to better cope with them and establish healthy ways to experience a wide variety of emotions, both good and bad. Using an emotional meter to assess your level of emotional need will give you the clarity you need to determine the next steps.

Even if you're feeling a-ok emotionally, it's wise to purposefully take actions to maintain a good balance. Individuals who are regularly solid can fill their spirits by sharing strategies with others to be a support to those around them. When you're in this stage of maintenance, it's a perfect time to consider routines you can add to your life that will sustain your emotional health and prevent yourself from getting emotionally drained.

The strain felt by emotions is powerful. Depression affects over 18 million adults and, when untreated, can have devastating effects. According to the National Network of Depression Centers, two-thirds of people with depression do not seek proper treatment. This is saddening because four out of five people who did receive treatment for depression experienced an improvement in depression-related symptoms in just four to six weeks.

Less severe cases of emotional drain can be addressed by boosting your mood with an emotional deposit or flooding your life with emotional care through the establishment of habits that benefit your emotional well-being. Preparing for events that you anticipate will weigh on you emotionally can help reduce how much you are drained. For example, if you and your sister-in-law frequently spar at family functions and you're likely to see her at your nephew's birthday party this weekend, you might have a code word with your partner to "save" you from the conflict. If that doesn't set you more at ease, another option might be using a broken-record strategy. When the conversation seems to escalate, plan to squash it by saying, "We might not agree on this topic, but I'm sure we can agree that our nephew is growing up fast."

Knowing you have a lifeline or a plan to change the subject is likely to keep your anxiousness down going into the party. With a more relaxed feeling, you might not be so quick to shift a conversation into a full-blown argument.

Identify, plan for, and respond to emotional stress to tend to this important area of your overall wellness. Your commitment to emotional strength doesn't mean you put on a happy face when you're not happy. It means recognizing the feelings you have, allowing yourself to feel a range of emotions, and taking action if you are emotionally unhealthy. Outline the steps you plan to take

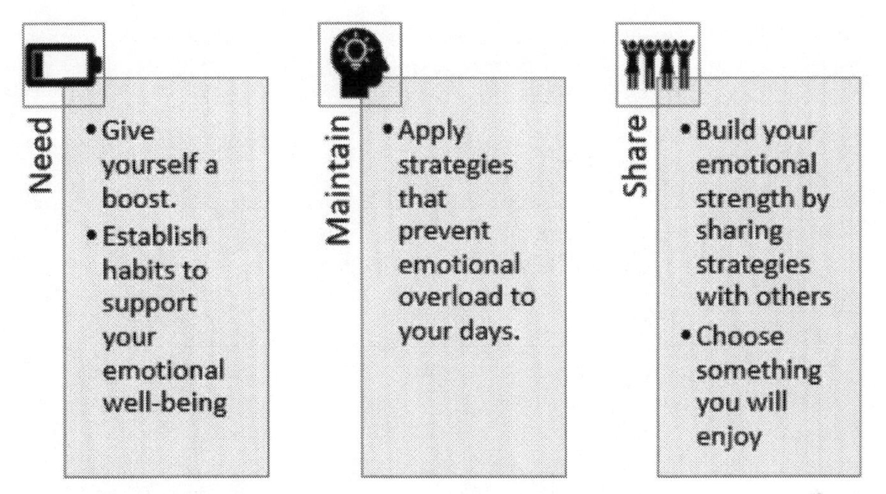

Figure 2.2: Emotional Meter Assessment. *Source:* Connie Hamilton

to build, maintain, feed, embed, and share emotional wellness (see Figure 2.2). Use the reflection questions to guide you.

1. How will you build habits that support your emotional wellness?
2. What will you do to maintain a healthy emotional self?
3. When necessary, what are some quick boosts to feed your emotional needs?
4. How can you care for your emotional self within the school day?
5. In what ways might you share or model the importance of emotional well-being with others?

Chapter 3

Devotion to Cognitive Care

Many philosophers, going all the way back to Marcus Aurelius in 180 AD, have noted that happiness comes from within. This means you cannot rely on external objects or powers to feed your soul with what you need. These opportunities must be created through self-care, which includes attending to your brain's need for exercise. In order to live your life as a forever learner, it will require you to challenge your cognition with difficult, yet doable tasks, and remove barriers that detract from your focus and concentration.

CEREBRAL FITNESS

Your brain is similar to the muscles in your body; if you fail to give it a workout, you can lose your ability to use it (Amen, 2012). Chapter 1 focused on using other muscles in the body to support physical well-being. Exercising your brain is equally as important as your triceps and heart. Additionally, giving yourself a cognitive workout promotes cerebral wellness. Teachers make a living training, flexing, and growing students' brains. However, when it comes to exercising their own brains, many educators do not reap the benefits that brain fitness provides in terms of their own happiness.

When they hear the words "school mental health," many think of the wellness of students, but school mental health also includes promoting the well-being of the adults within the school. The World Health Organization defines mental wellness as "a state of well-being in which the individual realizes his or her own abilities, can cope with the normal stresses of life, can work productively and fruitfully, and is able to make a contribution to his or her community" (Galderisi et al., 2015).

This is the very reason many teachers are drawn to education in the first place. They desire the opportunity to use their talents to tackle the challenges of educating today's youth to make our world and future a better place.

The centerpiece of professional growth for teachers has often been limited to offering professional development with little attention to the mental readiness teachers have to new learning. The common practice for delivering professional development is to just deliver it. Little or no regard given to the brain capacity the teachers have on any given professional development day.

Schools are not the only organizations that avoid the topic of their employees' mental health, because the topic of mental health is often misunderstood. Stigmas from lack of understanding are often attached to mental health, and attending to mental health issues can be seen by some as a weakness. The tendency of avoidance around this important subject is not helping anyone, especially teachers who are dealing with the stress of teaching, student trauma, parent demands, evaluation, and more.

To ensure your cognitive health needs are met, attend to conditions that embrace your ability to focus, concentrate, and be creative and take action to ward off those that hinder them. Healthy habits give the mind exercise, just like the body, to cultivate positive brain health. Cognitive self-care is engaging in any information to encourage stimulation of your mind and intellect.

In this chapter, you will explore different concepts and strategies to enhance your life and help make cognitive self-care part of your daily routine. To maximize your learning, there are the guiding questions for you to review. As you start this chapter, please reflect on the launch questions provided. The end of the chapter will offer after-reading reflection questions to guide you through processing the information provided and how it connects to your personal cognitive wellness.

1. What is my current definition of cognitive wellness?
2. How do I tend to my cognitive well-being?
3. What perception do I have of cognitive health?
4. What is something I hope to learn as I read?
5. How would I rate my current cognitive well-being barometer?

Allow your brain to work at its greatest potential by removing distractions. Some of these barriers include those discussed in chapters 1 and 2: lack of sleep, low self-esteem, and various kinds of stress all impact your ability to focus and think clearly. In other words, you cannot be at your cognitive best when you are not caring for all facets of your own well-being.

There is usually agreement among educators that the mental stimulation of students is important for the whole child. But if asked how they are planning for their own cognitive nurturing, the expected response is the sound of crickets. Nourishing your academic appetite means you are engaging in tasks that fall in the sweet spot of ease and difficulty. Teachers feel way too busy, and the idea of brain stimulation to care for their cognitive needs seems to be off their radars.

Teachers put the needs of others first: students, friends, family, coworkers, and simply anyone else appears to move up on the priority ladder, causing their own needs to be neglected. They find themselves taking on extra jobs at school when asked, staying late for what is presented to be a quick meeting, assisting with one more event, or tutoring one more child. The "yes" comes before considering the drain on their mental capacity. Then the spiral begins. Overcommitting leads to a lack of sleep, depleting the physical well-being container. The tiredness creates a barrier to thinking agility and cognitive well-being is also jeopardized.

As a teacher, it may feel selfish to put yourself first, but you must tend to your own needs to be at your cognitive best. Consider this your official permission to prioritize yourself and take care of your brain. Teaching is complex and requires significant cerebral agility. Just because you might have the time to add another commitment to your schedule doesn't mean you will have the cognitive capacity to put your brain in overdrive.

Perhaps an alternate perspective is to weigh the cost/benefit of tackling another project. Maybe prepping materials and setting up for the morning will give you more cognitive freedom later in the evening, permitting you to enjoy a challenging game of Sudoku. However, beware of the reverse effect. It's possible that signing up for one more committee will prevent you from having the time to join a wine club you and your partner have been wanting to enjoy.

Educators often pay more attention to the level of their phone battery than the level of their cognitive wellness. If the battery is too low, there is an urgency to quickly plug in the phone to charge the battery so there is optimum usage. Yet, if brain energy feels low, the instinct is often to forge through ignoring the need to recharge. Why is that?

Throughout this chapter, you will find various research-based cognitive wellness strategies that can be useful for you to incorporate into your routine. Take notes on the areas of self-care you would like to integrate into your schedule. Every person is unique, so focus on strategies that will work well for you. There will be time for reflection at the end of each section so you can dig deeper into your thoughts about each idea.

DAILY NOURISHMENT OF YOUR COGNITIVE WELLNESS

Establishing habits that make cognitive well-being part of your everyday routine doesn't have to drain your other self-care needs by taking too much time or forcing you to forego other important areas to provide balance. Consider how you might reap two or more benefits out of a single task or manage time more efficiently to open up your agenda. Bring intentional learning into your daily routine. The keyword is routine. Here are some easy ways to put your brain stretching on a schedule.

Word of the Day

Maybe you have a word of the day calendar that introduces you to one vocabulary word each day. Find a place to keep your calendar to view at some point in your morning. It could be on your bathroom wall, in your car, near the breakfast table, or on your desk. Each day rip off a sheet to reveal a word. Challenge yourself to find an opportunity to use the word before you go to sleep. There are also free online subscriptions that will send a dictionary word to your email each day. This is a great alternative for those teachers who prefer to use their technology.

D.E.A.R.

Yes, this refers to the good ol' "Drop Everything and Read" time. Only this time you do the reading. Whether you choose to read a book for pleasure or you are dedicated to checking in on a daily blog, the point is to bring learning through reading into your everyday norm. Better yet, consider a book that helps you lift another area of wellness, like how to save time and money. That way you will be elevating two needs at once.

Reading books is beneficial for your mental health, and the benefits can last a lifetime (Stanborough, 2019). Reading a book is a simple way to improve your mood. Commit to reading something of interest for 30 minutes a day. Reading for pleasure has many benefits and can result in improved relationships, increased empathy, improved well-being, and reduction in symptoms of depression and dementia (Reading Agency, 2015).

Listen and Learn

Today there are more ways than ever to absorb content. Reading is one way, but you might choose to use your ears to soak up information or entertainment. Podcasts and audiobooks make it easy to digest on the move. Instead of listening to the radio the entire drive to work, try plugging into a podcast that talks about cooking or teaching. You will be surprised how much you can glean in a short amount of time. Other great opportunities for listening include walking the dog, doing household chores, or saving 15 minutes before bed to lay down, relax, and power up your brain's battery.

Take Micro-Breaks

It's true that the brain needs activity to keep it sharp and functioning efficiently. It also needs rest. Studies found that detaching from work either physically or through relaxation is associated with a lower need for long recoveries (Coffeng et al., 2015). Research has also found that these breaks can reduce stress and help keep you productive throughout your day. A short walk down the hall, a stretch break, or a mindful moment are all examples of micro-breaks that can give your mind a reboot it needs.

Sign Up for a Club

Check out your community's social media pages to see what opportunities exist for you to join a club. Some options might include parenting groups, book clubs, or groups that provide a community service focus like a group that volunteers at a local hospital or educates the community on a cause that is important to you. Try to focus on areas of your life outside education. Your identity as a teacher is key, but it doesn't define you. Feed your mental muscle by expanding an interest or hobby that will offer you cognitive challenge, a sense of accomplishment, joy, and a break from the job.

Maximize Your Calendar

An organized calendar and subsequently, time simplifies your life and helps you feel more in control. Schedule time for planning lessons in your calendar to help you focus on a time to plan and eliminate procrastination. Make use of an online platform such as planbook.com to help keep your lesson plans organized and easily accessible.

Launch Reminders on Your Phone

Many educators use Google Calendar to keep a schedule; this will allow them to share or partially share their calendars with others. If you are not using this tool yet, pick a calendar app that works for you. A human resource director that Dorothy worked with kept track of everything on her phone but wanted a paper copy of her calendar to see each day. She found it helpful to print out her calendar instead of looking at her phone.

Batch Tasks

Just because you're invited to a meeting or committee, doesn't always mean you have to say yes. Jostling different tasks throughout the day is inefficient.

Consider each meeting invite and request; if it's something you will be adding to your calendar, be the first to suggest a time based on what is most convenient and productive for you.

Begin to group similar activities together in your calendar. If you need to give written feedback to students and prep materials for the next unit, schedule time in your calendar to block out time for these tasks. If you need to make five parent calls and six parent emails, batch these tasks together on your calendar and complete them in a single chunk of time. You will get more accomplished if you do all the communication in an allocated time, rather than spreading it out over the week and worrying about it each day that you still need to complete the task.

Consistency Is Key

Keep a consistent routine in your schedule, this includes going to bed and waking up at similar times each night and day. Put everything into your calendar, even things like a playdate with your kids or grocery shopping. Allocating time for all your events and required tasks will give you a better picture of what time you have available. This prevents overcommitting or foregoing something you hoped to do but scheduled something else in its place.

Color It

Color-code your calendar to make it visually easy to see what categories and descriptions you have organized. Each color can represent a different category: orange can be for school tasks, green for personal activities, and blue for self-care time. As you become comfortable with color-coding, you may wish to add more categories.

Reminders and Tasks

Use reminder tools to help you keep track of upcoming events. If you have a big project that has to be done by October 15, set a reminder the week before "Project due in one week" so it doesn't sneak up on you.

Break Up

Make challenging goals manageable by breaking them into chunks. Take a calendar for the year and break it down into quarters, so you will have four three-month sections. Now, break your goal into these quarters. Write out the big ideas that you will need to accomplish each quarter to achieve this goal.

Next, take each quarter and break it into months and again, assign pieces of your big ideas to each month.

Now, a year-long goal is segmented and less overwhelming. Once you feel comfortable with what you will be doing each month for your goal, break the months down into weeks. This strategy will take you from a 30,000-foot view of your goal to more manageable steps.

Host Your Own Blog

Teachers love to share and receive tips and tools from one another. Why not start a blog that narrates some of your successes and describes challenges you are having in the classroom? You might be surprised by how therapeutic it is to have a channel to connect with others. If you commit to posting on a schedule, you will soon find that writing becomes part of your reflection and style of processing.

If you don't want to blog about education, consider blogging about something else. One of the most interesting blogs Connie enjoyed reading was a homeowner who shared posts as her house was being built. It was helpful to read what could be expected, how to prepare, and what pitfalls to avoid.

You can literally blog about *anything*! Other ideas include blogging about parenting, gardening, vacationing, or your thoughts about a favorite TV show. The topic is less important than the mental benefits you'll gain by sharing, letting go of the immediate tasks, and homing in on your interest. Chapters 4 and 5 will talk about social and spiritual well-being. A blog can be a great way to tend to a trifecta of benefits for you.

This Is How We Do It

A major benefit of establishing routines is that it provides a sense of security for everyone. Routines play a significant role in mental health (Arlinghaus & Johnston, 2018) and can help manage stress and anxiety (Eilam, et al., 2011). Children and adults feel more confident and secure when their schedule is predictable and familiar.

Start with the most troublesome tasks in your home. Bedtime? Meal prep? Homework? Household chores? Think of the task as a flow chart. What happens first? Then what? What's the very last step? Don't take on too much; one routine is enough to feel an impact. Communicate to all the stakeholders what the routine is and what their role is in its execution.

Take meal prep, for example. Maybe one child is tasked with setting the table, someone preps the meal, a chef's assistant handles ongoing clean-up while cooking and manages multiple tasks that need to happen quickly. Then someone else can be assigned to clean the table. If you want to be even more specific, you can get very detailed. Choose one table cleaner to move dirty dishes near the sink while another table cleaner puts condiments away and packs up any leftovers.

Whatever you decide, stick to it. After the task is done, debrief. Who did what job? How did it go? Any adjustments we need to make? Then celebrate your success. Preferably with something fun for everyone—including YOU. Sit at your clean table or in the eyesight of your tidy kitchen and designate five minutes for each person to share the highlight of their day or something they're looking forward to the next day. Not only will you be establishing a routine to get a necessary task completed, but you'll be enjoying the benefit of freeing up time to fill another self-care bucket, all while modeling great habits for the rest of your family.

WHEN YOU NEED A COGNITIVE BOOST

When you recognize that you're not giving your brain what it needs to maintain balance, you might consider a single event to ramp up your mental capacity. When choosing an approach to boost your cognitive well-being, consider ways you can get in a flow. "Research finds that people are happiest when engaged in difficult-but-doable activities," writes Laura Vanderkam in *Fortune* (Rampton, 2017).

Charles Limb, a neuroscientist at Johns Hopkins, studied Csikszentmihalyi's flow (see Figure 3.1). He found that when jazz musicians were in flow, the dorsolateral prefrontal cortex disengaged (Kotler, 2017). This is the area of the brain that is responsible for self-monitoring. It is the little voice in your

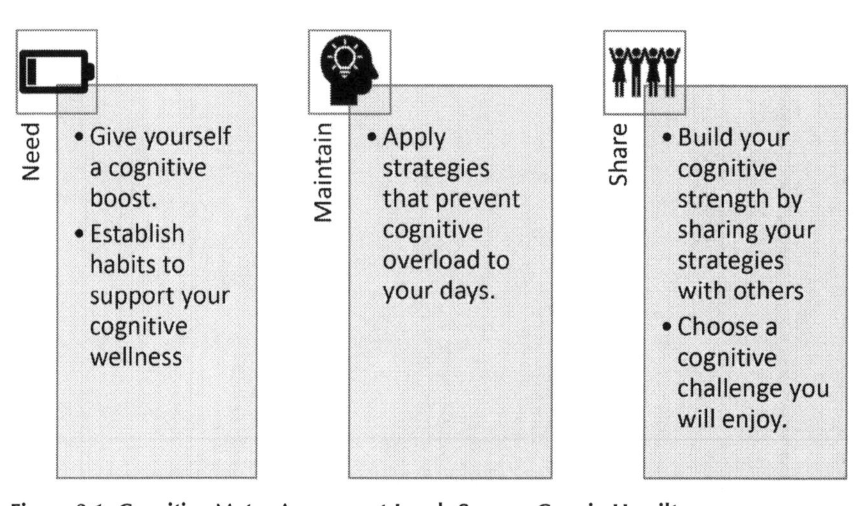

Figure 3.1: Cognitive Meter Assessment Level. ***Source:*** **Connie Hamilton**

head that questions your choices and slows your decisions. When this part of the brain is quieted, the outcome is liberation. The fear of failure dissipates, and there is a sort of automaticity that is described by many.

Flow falls in the sweet spot between boredom when a task is too easy for someone's skill level and anxiety when the task is too difficult. Brain studies suggest that we are in a daydream-like state where things seem to flow without hesitation. It isn't just jazz musicians who experience flow. If you've ever said to yourself or someone else "I don't want to stop, I'm on a roll," you might have been in flow.

In these peaks, you are so engrossed in your project or task that your sense of time is lost and you're able to turn off other thoughts that might otherwise flood your head. Activities, projects, or adventures that help you get in the *flow* increase your happiness. Perhaps this is where the common idiom "time flies when you're having fun" is scientifically connected.

Browse the following ideas that might help you to get into a flow. When you land on one that appeals to you, give it a try. If the list inspires a different idea, run with it.

Tackle a Project

Big or small, completing a project is not only gratifying, but it will give you a shot of cognitive boost that you might be needing. The benefits of restaining a table or waxing your car include a mental break from stresses you might not be able to put to rest. Redirecting your attention to something that requires focus will make you feel productive and give your head a cognitive reboot.

Declutter or Organize

Clutter and disorganization can have a negative effect on our mental health. Tidy up your space. Not only will your area be cleaner, but your brain also performs better when things are organized (Klemm, 2016). Setting personal and professional goals provide a clear focus and a sense of purpose. At home, decide which area you will organize, set aside an hour, determine a day, and then get to work straightening up the designated space. Make this enjoyable by turning on some music and grabbing a refreshing drink. You may organize alone or enlist family members to help.

At work, think about the space in your classroom that needs organization. Allocate a date and time limit to clean up the space. This may be a task to conquer yourself, or include students to build ownership and model respect for the classroom and the things in it. One strategy is to separate items into three areas; trash, recycle, and donation. In the case of donation of classroom items, you may be able to give these items to another staff member, so be sure to check with fellow colleagues to see if they can use the items before you take them to a donation center.

Disorganization can be anywhere; consider these spaces and determine if decluttering will improve your ability to know where things are and quickly access what you need. When spaces are organized in a logical way, you will be able to reserve your cognitive energy for more enjoyable things than "Where can I find a postage stamp?" Some ideas for organizational consideration include:

- Dedicate a weekend to sort through old photos. You will likely enjoy the mental trip down memory lane, and you'll gain peace of mind that your precious pictures are safe and organized.
- Visit your kitchen pantry to identify donations for a local food pantry and make your items easy to access.
- Throw out expired or unused medication in your bathroom cabinet.
- Create a system for keeping track of tax documents.
- Sanitize toys in your child's toy box and remove any broken or outgrown toys.
- Split overgrown plants in your yard and offer the extras to neighbors through social media channels.
- Sort your classroom book collection. Label or re-shelve books by genre, reading level, or theme.

Tap into Your Inner Artist

Have fun expressing yourself artistically as you stimulate other learning. Jensen states in *Arts with the Brain in Mind* (2001, p. 3), "The systems they nourish, which include our integrated sensory, attentional, cognitive, emotional, and motor capacities, are, in fact, the driving forces behind all other learning." This means that triggering your creative juices feeds other brain functions that impact your mental skills. Here are some ideas to get your thinking about how to express yourself.

- Create a piece of abstract art and save it for a family member's birthday gift.
- Join your teen in creating a TikTok video.
- Write a poem and dedicate it to a loved one.
- Write a five-minute stand-up routine and host a comedy night at your house.

Game Night

You likely have a cabinet of educational games in your classroom. Games can activate creativity, critical thinking, and fun. Your brain will enjoy a break from routine when you bring out the Scrabble board or choose something less cognitively straining like Jenga. If you feel like stimulating the mind solo, select one-player games such as solitaire, Sudoku, or Bananagrams.

BELL-TO-BELL DEVOTION TO COGNITIVE CARE

As noted in the introduction, teaching is one of the most stressful professions in America today. Therefore, it is even more crucial that educators can identify the symptoms of increasing stress and initiate coping skills to manage it. Unfortunately, teachers do not have the luxury of being able to respond immediately when their bodies and minds are reaching their maximum stress.

Decreased mental sharpness, shortened attention span, reduced patience, fatigue, and even physical pain are all indications of mental exhaustion (Santos-Longhurst, 2018). Preventative practices and a backpack of reactive strategies that can reduce your cognitive load are ways to combat mental fatigue.

On the other hand, keeping your mind challenged and processing information gives you the academic exercise needed to have a strong brain functioning. A balance of cognitive challenge and rest throughout the day will keep your thinking agile. Consider these strategies that are designed to address your cognitive needs that boost thinking and mental processing. They offer opportunities to tend to an overstressed head during the school days.

Maintain the Why

Sometimes your groove might become mundane. Mentally exhausted teachers can go through the motions of facilitating learning without a keen focus on why a particular strategy is being used. It's easier than dismissing the strategy as ineffective when the anticipated outcome misaligns with the actual results. When implementing best instructional practices, keep a cognitive focus on the purpose of the activity.

Is the intent for a think-pair-share to maintain a quiet environment or is it designed to give students an opportunity to verbally process their thinking? If, after this commonly used strategy, students are still struggling to understand, direct your reflection on the learning routine. Did students have enough think -time before being prompted to pair and share? Are students partnered in a way that feels safe to them? Is your determination of success based on a single student's response?

Freshen Up

Sometimes a fresh approach is just what is needed to give yourself a cognitive boost and spark creativity. Try rearranging your classroom or reversing your classroom agenda. Maybe you want to try a new strategy you read about on a blog. A shake-up now and then, especially when you plan it, can be all it takes to get those brain juices flowing again. Of course, change isn't viewed as refreshing to everyone, so use this tip if you're feeling the need for a little change.

Dedicate Time to Problem-Solving Issues That Require Strategic Thinking

One thing Dorothy and Connie have learned in their own careers is that not every problem needs to be solved right now. Of course, if a student has a health emergency, it doesn't make sense to pause and pull out a journal to process the best course of action. There are times when it's necessary to quickly make a decision and respond swiftly.

However, when it comes right down to it, very few of the most important decisions teachers make each day are time-sensitive. Consider reserving the more complex problems for a time when you can pull all of your cognitive attention together and direct it to find the best solutions. You are more likely to gain clarity when you aren't monitoring a classroom of students asking for support on their project-based learning task.

Bring Routines to the Classroom

As suggested in the "Daily Nourishment of Your Cognitive Wellness" section of this chapter, instituting routines for yourself is one of the habits suggested to free your mind. The automaticity of a routine frees space for thinking and focusing on deeper learning. These routines are beneficial for students too. Establishing that consistency and completing tasks in the same order frequently builds brain power and supports cognitive health (Miller, 2017).

When your classroom doesn't feel like a three-ring circus, you can focus your attention on more important teacher tasks like formative assessment and quality feedback rather than spending your mental energy on classroom management.

Keep Your Classroom Neat

You've heard the phrase "A tidy space indicates a tidy mind." Well, it turns out there is some neurological truth to it. According to a study by Princeton Neuroscience Institute, your brain has a maximum amount of stimuli that it can process (McMains & Kastner, 2011). Excessive visuals within a person's view cause competition in the brain for where your brain's attention will be drawn.

This competition reduces the ability or level of focus you have on a cognitive task. Therefore, when your vision is free of chaotic scenery, you can dedicate more attention to your thoughts without distraction from images in the room. By the way, this also applies to students, so use classroom decorations sparingly and go for an orderly and purposeful look to keep students and you focused on more important things than wall decorations.

Brain Breaks

Spontaneous and scheduled brain breaks definitely have their place in your day. Use spontaneous breaks when you're getting foggy or find concentrating a challenge.

When you schedule plans for a break, be mindful of how you are spending that time. Do you need to solve a problem? Is this a break moment to do it?- Or has it been "one of those days" and a brief distraction is more beneficial? Remember, these are brief.

- Count student heads—it allows you to keep your eye on the students and build in a half-minute to reset.
- Lap the class—if you find yourself stuck in one spot, move from that position and visit all corners of the classroom.
- Play soft music—it allows you to get up and moving and provides a mental distraction when you need one.
- Have a student fill in—students can't always lead the class, but often there are tasks such as reading directions or selecting volunteers they can handle. If a student can take the lead, even for a minute, it will free you up to rest your mind or direct your focus to something more pressing.

If you need more than a minute or so, look for ways to give yourself the reprieve you need. It's true that there isn't much time from bell to bell for a mental vacation to reboot. That's why having strategies like these in mind can make the difference between being drained all day or tending to your cognitive needs so you can cope with the strains that teaching demands.

Brain Break with the Entire Class

If you're needing a cognitive pause, it's possible your students do too. Bring in box breathing, a wiggle release, or shift to a brief share session of good news. There are countless activities and ideas to invite your class to a brain break with you.

Actually Break When You Break

It is a given that time is scarce during the school day. However, it's important to take advantage of the few opportunities you have to take a short mental vacation. It's suggested to sing the alphabet when you wash your hands—try singing it backward. Not only will it take a little longer, but it's also likely to pull your brain away from everything that might be spinning around—even two minutes.

Chitchat

During lunch, spend time socializing with other teachers and keep the conversation light and positive. There will be more on the benefits of socialization in chapter 4.

SHARE YOUR COGNITIVE THINKING

Once your self-care needs are met, you may find yourself seeking opportunities to optimize your knowledge. With your cerebral backpack filled with strategies to combat mental strain or drain in the form of exhaustion or boredom, you're well on your way to a cognitively healthier you. With a balance of challenge and rest for your brain, you might be in a place to share your successful approaches with others. In doing so, you will be multiplying the benefits you get for yourself. Sharing with others supports social wellness that will be discussed more in the next chapter.

Depending on the activity, you can also add to any physical or emotional needs. Offer to help someone set up for a party. They will get some mental relief knowing you're there to help, and you will reap the emotional benefit of providing an act of service. And if that's not enough, there are social buckets being filled. Cognitive, emotional, and social needs met with a single task? Hot diggity! Here are some brainstormed options for you to share your brain power and help lift others.

Start a Book Club

Maybe you have an interest or know someone who has one. Starting a book club will increase the likelihood that you will finally dig in. Leading the group reduces the cognitive burden on others who participate while giving them an opportunity to feed their brains. The benefit of a book club versus reading a book on your own is the dialogue that occurs when readers are understanding a new idea or making connections in different ways. The social aspect of the book club encourages members to read more and gives more confidence in professional discussions (Coleman, 2016).

Present at a Workshop or Conference

As educators who have presented hundreds of times to thousands of educators, we still find it surprising how many teachers underestimate the interest others have in their experience and knowledge. Sharing your success by organizing peer coaching sessions or describing how you walked through steps to create a podcast run by students are examples of topics that would pack a room of teachers wanting more information. If you're a bit reticent about presenting to your peers, invite a coworker to present with you. This will split the work and give you the confidence you need.

Mentor Another Teacher

The traditional view of the most experienced teacher being assigned a newbie as a mentee is not the only structure for successful mentoring. In their book, *Modern Mentor*, Brooks and Joseph (2019) describe a partnership where veteran teachers learn a specific skill or strategy from a teacher with a shorter resume. This pairing is mutually beneficial. If you are a lesson-experienced teacher with an area of expertise, collaborating with a more seasoned teacher will not only help them learn a new skill, but you're likely to pick up a few tricks of the trade as well.

Donate Unused or Unwanted Clothing

Purging your wardrobe contributes to others in a different way. You gain the benefit of decluttering your closet and dresser drawers and someone else gets the opportunity for a spiffy new outfit or much-needed clothing. If you're feeling especially ambitious, add a step by bringing your clothes basket to a second-hand shop that buys back used clothing. Give them the first pick of your items, then take what they pass on to a donation center. Here's a project that literally pays off!

FEATURE THE TEACHER WITH COGNITIVE WELLNESS

Mrs. Mueller never had an interest in sewing, but her husband thought she might enjoy the idea so he bought her a sewing machine as a gift in 2002 when she was a young teacher. Trying to make the best of her new present, she learned how to sew and began making some blankets for her own children and for gifts. Ironically, her sister, Mrs. Chatfield—also a teacher—was an avid sewer and would encourage her to try new patterns.

One day, while shopping together, they saw a very expensive hooded towel at a small boutique, and her sister purchased the towel. Mrs. Chatfield was determined to make these beautiful towels. Sure enough, she figured out how to make the hooded towels and quickly taught Mrs. Mueller how to make them as well. In the classroom, Mrs. Mueller often thought about how learning from her sister bonded them and grew their relationship. She strived to provide that same sense of partnership as she taught her students new things.

When sewing, Mrs. Mueller found her thoughts drifting away as she laughed and developed her sewing skills. When friends or family had a baby, Mrs. Mueller and Mrs. Chatfield would give a homemade hooded towel as a present. Over time, their hooded towel gifts became more popular and soon, friends and family started requesting some of her creations.

What started as a hobby slowly turned into a small business. They started selling the towels at craft shows, and over time orders would pour in from across the county. The extra income Mrs. Mueller earned from her sewing business funded her daughter's dance lessons and expenses. The hobby came full circle during the pandemic of 2020; Mrs. Mueller started sewing homemade masks with the extra fabric scraps and she donated hundreds of them to health care workers and teachers.

Mrs. Mueller shares this experience with students. It's particularly relevant when students are facing something that is completely new to them. She encourages an open mind and willingness to explore new things. You never know, today's lesson could pave the way for a student's future career.

EDUCATOR COMMITMENT TO COGNITIVE CARE

Before developing your plan to address your cognitive fitness, use these end-of-chapter questions to metacognitively consider what you're understanding about your cognitive care.

1. How has my definition of cognitive wellness been confirmed or shifted?
2. What new perspectives have I gained about cognitive health?

3. What are some ways I can intentionally build my cognitive well-being?
4. What new learning have I acquired?

Now, apply your understanding of cognitive wellness from this chapter to your own self-care. Table 3.1 provides some reflection statements to help with a needs assessment.
Choose your favorite reflection process to review your responses to Table 3.1. Revisit the checklist from time to time. It will likely change over time based on your attention to yourself and the events that occur in your life and your classroom. Get a snapshot of where your cognitive wellness is. Using a three-column process, enter the date in the first column and mindfully describe your cognitive status. What seems to be influencing your overall wellness in this area? Here is a sample entry:

January 5: The break from school and seeing family was energizing. Getting back into a routine after the holidays has helped me stay focused.

Now that you have collected a snapshot, look ahead to what might put a cognitive strain on you. For example:

The new semester begins soon. I will be teaching a new class, so I have a lot to figure out in the next few weeks.

Take your checklist and snapshots into consideration. Based on your needs assessment reflection, choose where you are on the mental meter in Figure 3.1. There is not a formula that places you in a specific box. Everyone is different, so you have to determine what's best for you.

If you find yourself falling in the "Need" category of the mental meter assessment level, we suggest you give yourself a cognitive boost and use the momentum you gain to begin working to develop habits that build cognitive well-being into your everyday life. If your assessment lands you in the "Maintain" category, your goal is to keep it there. Adding preventative strategies to your wellness backpack will help you avoid overload and the risk of falling back into the need category.

When your reflection provides you with confidence that your cognitive well-being is solid, you can place yourself in the "Share" category. When you're at this level, we cautiously recommend you continue to build your strength by sharing coping strategies with others or inviting them to join you on some of your favorite ways you tend to your cognitive needs.

The amount of mental exertion you have will vary from day to day, even minute to minute. Some strains on your mind will last moments and others might carry on for weeks. This is common, but it doesn't mean you have

Table 3.1: Cognitive Care Needs Assessment Checklist

	Never/ Rarely	Occasionally	Frequently/ Always
I have difficulty concentrating on tasks.			
I am easily distracted.			
I feel overwhelmed by what I have to learn.			
My mental exhaustion impedes my productivity.			
My brain feels stretched to the maximum.			
I feel like I need a cognitive break.			
I have trouble getting into a "flow."			
I enjoy tasks or games that challenge my thinking.			
When given a puzzle, I am determined to solve it.			
I love to learn new things.			
My interests outside school require brain power.			
I focus better in a clutter-free environment.			
I bet bored when things are the same.			
I make decisions without thinking them through.			
I have difficulty multitasking.			
My knowledge is underutilized.			
I intentionally tend to my cognitive wellness.			
I can recognize when I need a cognitive boost.			
My cognitive care backpack has strategies that help me in this area of wellness.			

to jeopardize your overall well-being because your brain is being taxed. If events that will require heavy thinking can be anticipated, such as a day set aside for student data analysis or a paper due in your master's class, you can prepare.

The concept of deposits and withdrawals we shared in chapter 2 can be used to think about your cognitive capacity as well. Some things are going to drain your cognitive bank more rapidly than others. To avoid a deficit, which will result in irritability, fatigue, and inability to concentrate, you can purposefully take action to keep some cerebral juice in your tank.

Create a T-chart and label one side "withdrawal cognitive energy" and the other side "self-care response." Use your entries to view what is pulling on you at school and determine how to offset it. The same chart can be used for various parts of your life that may be impacting your mental load such as family, home, or planning a big event like a graduation party.

Now, you're ready to make a commitment to your cognitive fitness. Use what you have learned in this chapter about establishing habits, providing cognitive boosts, and including self-care from bell to bell. Identify the strategies you want to start implementing to improve your cognitive fitness, actions within your control that you need to stop doing because they are draining your brain, and strategies that seem to be working and you should continue to use. Use the guiding questions to help you.

1. How will you build habits that support your cognitive wellness?
2. What will you do to maintain a healthy cognitive self?
3. When necessary, what are some quick boosts to feed your cognitive needs?
4. How can you care for your cognitive wellness within the school day?
5. In what ways might you share or model the importance of cognitive well-being with others?

Chapter 4

Concentration on Social Prosperity

In education, the student-teacher relationship is not only valued, it's often a school or district focus to find ways to help students connect to peers and staff. The same commitment to building connections among adults is often forgotten or unaddressed. According to Brené Brown, connection is why we are here as a species. Brown's (2015) research shows we are hardwired to connect with others; it is what gives purpose and meaning to our lives. Without connection there is suffering.

This doesn't mean you have to become a social butterfly if you're not as comfortable in large groups as others. It does mean that social interactions have an impact on your overall well-being, and all of us can benefit in one way or another by socializing with others. This chapter will help you determine ways to maximize your relationships and interactions with others so your social connections will elevate your overall wellness.

Do you classify yourself as an extrovert because you are comfortable in social settings and have close and meaningful friendships? Or maybe you self-label as an introvert because you are not confident speaking in front of peers or are considered to be sensitive. Well, you might be wrong. The difference between extroversion or introversion is commonly overgeneralized as extroverts being people who are confident and those who are quiet are deemed introverts. *Confident* and *quiet* are emotions, and at times, are felt by everyone. But being an introvert or extrovert isn't connected to your emotions. Even dictionaries and thesauruses misconstrue extroverts as being outgoing, gregarious, and friendly while describing introverts as aloof, shy, or withdrawn. Turns out, none of that is accurate.

Psychologists don't see people as being either extroverts or introverts. According to Carl Jung, a psychologist who is credited with creating the psychological concept of extroversion and introversion, they are viewed more on a continuum (Houston, 2021). This means everyone has tendencies for both. When one side of the spectrum is more dominant than the other, that's when someone is considered an introvert or extrovert. Those who fall smack dab in the middle are called *ambiverts*.

Whether you are an introvert or an extrovert depends on two things. First, how you create energy and second, how you process information. Introverts look internally to build energy and make sense of the world while extroverts seek out others to recharge and process information on the fly, often verbally. As an introvert, you might be the life of the party and comfortable in public. Then after a social event, crash as soon as you're alone, exhausted by the energy it takes to keep up in a social setting. Conversely, extroverts tend to refuel when they are with others and might even have trouble winding down when the crowd goes home because they have harnessed so much energy from others.

What's relevant to knowing where you fall on the introvert/extrovert scale is that it allows you to make sure that you allocate time to recharge in a way that is going to maximize your energy boost. If sharing your success with someone motivates you, then as an extrovert, it will be helpful to have someone or some way to communicate your progress to keep up your momentum. On the other hand, if you're more introverted and have a collaboration session to attend, it will be helpful for you to prepare by first reflecting on your own so you have gathered your thoughts and feel ready to benefit from the group work session. Tending to your needs will help you get the most out of social interactions and keep you energized.

Introverts and extroverts alike benefit from socializing. This chapter is dedicated to helping you find ways to connect with others and intentionally select actions that will position you to be at your personal best. As you read through the chapter, look for strategies that speak to you and are likely to help you tend to your social needs.

Actions for introverts will likely be dissimilar to those for extroverts because they approach thinking and interaction in different ways. You will be able to identify ways to recharge based on your personality type. Introverts will gather tools to support them in social settings while extroverts will learn how to flourish even when alone. Ambiverts will find a mixture of strategies that provide the perfect balance for maximizing energy. This chapter is dedicated to help you find ways to connect with others and intentionally select actions that will position you to be at your personal best.

Review the following questions. Before you continue reading this chapter, consider the reflection prompts provided. This will help alert you to your current thoughts, feelings, and beliefs about your social well-being.

1. What is my current understanding of social wellness?
2. In what ways do I think my relationships, connections, and interactions impact my social wellness?

3. How do I tend to my social well-being?
4. What can I do to get the most out of my socializing?
5. What is something I hope to learn as I read about social wellness?
6. How would I rate my current social well-being barometer?

THE ROLE OF RELATIONSHIPS

Even though we live in a very social society with the ratio of extroverts to introverts being three to one (Cain, 2013), the goal isn't to turn everyone into an extrovert. It is also true that it is not helpful to isolate introverts and exclude them from social settings. A balanced life that offers just enough connection with others while providing sufficient time for just you varies from person to person. We all need both. However, how much we need depends on your neurodiversity.

In an interview with *Business Insider*, doctor of psychology Perpetua Neo shared that science comes into play when understanding how the brains of introverts and extroverts differ. Neo explained introverts are more sensitive to dopamine (Dodgson, 2018). As shared in chapter 2, dopamine is the chemical that makes you feel good when it's released. This heightened level of sensitivity causes introverts to be stimulated more easily, which can cause them to exert more energy to keep up with all that stimulation.

This explains why there is a feeling of exhaustion after particularly high levels of socialization. Neo explains, "So essentially what happens is after too much social stimulation, whether we're talking about small groups or a noisy overstimulated context, an introvert's nervous system is overwhelmed." The result is what is known as the *introvert hangover* or the need to unwind, typically alone. The calmness provides content, happiness, and replenishes the energy used after too much social stimulation.

Social interactions occur with strangers, acquaintances, colleagues, friends, family, and loved ones. In a recent study, researchers found that the strength of the participants' social circle was more related to their stress, happiness, and well-being than the health data collected on a fitness tracker (Lin et al., 2019). This demonstrates how important time with family and close friends is to your social and mental health. Whether you are an introvert or an extrovert, the benefits of spending social time with those closest to you is a critical component of a full and meaningful life.

Having an active social life produces many benefits including living a longer life, having better physical health, and improved mood and mental health (Ducharme, 2019). As you can see, tending to your social self-care directly impacts other areas of your individual wellness. Social well-being is the easiest piece of the whole teacher's self-care to double dip—meaning, a boost in any other category of wellness can be layered with a social benefit simply by doing it with a friend or loved one. Chapter 6 shares more details on the whole teacher's wellness.

Tending to your social self-care includes nurturing the relationships you already have, building healthy new relationships, and creating healthy boundaries to clearly communicate what expectations you have for others and what they can expect from you. This chapter highlights ways to establish habits that encourage you to make room for socializing while balancing other aspects of your life, how to use social settings to get a boost when you're feeling lonely or secluded, strategies that can be used to nurture your social well-being during the school day, and how you can support others to benefit from having quality relationships and engaging socially.

MAKING ROOM FOR BALANCED SOCIALIZATION

Developing habits that build, maintain, and manage relationships in your life not only helps you balance socialization, but offers a safety net for others to support your efforts to tend to your overall well-being. Thinking about how you grow and nurture your social circles permits you to make intentional decisions about how to expand your networks; enjoy family, friends, and loved ones; and reduce negative impacts others might have on your day or your emotional health.

The strategies in this section are offered to make social care part of your regular routine. As with any aspect of self-care, some of the ideas will feel easier and more fun to try out. However, push yourself to experiment with ideas that are good for your social wellness, even if you are not excited with the idea. Just like exercise and a balanced diet promotes your physical wellness, taking care of your social wellness might include activities that lead to good results although you may not be eager to engage in them.

Draw a Line

Establish boundaries with people in your life to honor yourself, communicate your needs, and set limits in a healthy way. The boundaries you establish with one person do not (and often are not) the same as others. For example, you might establish a physical boundary of space between you and a student when sitting next to each other during a small group. With a family member, you might be comfortable sitting so closely that your hips or arms are touching.

The setting might also impact your expectations. You may have a student who knows your family outside of school and calls you by your first name, but in the classroom you might prefer for them to use a salutation. You might have to clarify this distinction to your student. While boundaries should be somewhat flexible, that isn't a reason to not establish them at all.

Communicating your expectations with friends, colleagues, students, and others takes the mystery out of how interactions will take place. Healthy boundaries improve your relationships, and give you a sense of agency where you are aware of the needs you have in a relationship and appropriately share that with the other person. Conversely, a lack of boundaries can have people feeling disrespected or resentful. These thoughts about a relationship can deteriorate the connection and possibly break down or completely sever a relationship without the participants knowing why.

Although not all experts identify the same labels for types of boundaries, emotional, time, physical, intellectual, and material are some common categories recognized by many. Pause and think about how these types of boundaries play out in different settings. What boundaries do you have at home, in public, or at school? How do they change for family, students, coworkers, or people new to your circle?

Emotional Boundaries

Emotional boundaries respect feelings and energy related to how you and others are feeling. This means making sure someone is honoring your feelings or limiting how or what they are sharing with you. Some examples of how you communicate an emotional boundary include:

- When I open up to you in this way and you laugh or brush it off, it makes me feel like you aren't taking me seriously. If I share with you, I need you to try to relate to how I'm feeling without dismissing my emotions.
- It seems like this is an important topic and I'm not in the headspace to dedicate the energy it deserves today. Can we discuss this when I am able to focus better?
- I really need a caring ear right now. Is this a good time for us to talk?
- That's more than I'm comfortable sharing with you at this point. It's a little too personal.

Time Boundaries

Prioritizing how, where, and with whom you spend your time can be a challenge. Overcommitting to others diminishes the time you have for yourself and the autonomy to choose how and with whom you spend it. This can be especially prominent at school. When you have a grasp on where you want to spend your time and an awareness of how much time you have to offer to others, creating time boundaries helps you safeguard the precious minutes in your days. These examples might help you frame how you want to limit the time requested by others:

- I would love to attend, but I already have other plans at that same time.
- I'm happy to help, but I have a hard stop time of 4:30 pm.
- This week is already very busy. I'd prefer if we move it to next week when I have more time.
- When would be a good time for a 15-minute conversation I'd like to have with you?
- That sounds like a great idea, what kind of time commitment would I be making if I agree?

Physical Boundaries

Physical boundaries include touch, proximity, actions of affection, and your physical needs like sleep and food. They can also include comments about physical appearance or sexuality. Like many boundaries, culture, geographic region, personality types, family dynamics, and life experiences impact how people acknowledge personal space and physical boundaries. You can avoid awkward or uncomfortable situations by sharing your physical boundaries in a way that might sound something like:

- I need to take a break.
- That type of comment/joke is not welcomed by me.
- I have a bigger-than-average personal bubble, I am not comfortable when people stand so close to me.
- The invitation is tempting, but I need to get a good night's sleep. Can we do it another time?
- I'm more concerned with inner beauty than outward appearances.
- I prefer a handshake instead of a hug.
- No. You cannot touch me like that.

Intellectual Boundaries

Thoughts and ideas are often shared in social settings. Most everyone has a story about a time when they tried to share their thoughts with someone who has differing views. There are countless blogs, podcasts, and articles that warn of the three things you should never talk about—even with family. Politics. Religion. Money. Without establishing boundaries about how people will agree to disagree, topics like government can quickly sour a social interaction.

However, conversations about topics that some people find difficult or uncomfortable are necessary for us to make progress as a society. Topics like racism, for example, when discussed within intellectual boundaries can help people see alternate perspectives and maybe even shift others' beliefs. Here are some suggestions for how to request respectful ways to speak and listen to thoughts, ideas, or wonderings:

- This is a topic I am passionate about. Maybe we should choose a different time/location for this conversation.
- It seems that our discussion isn't leading us in a positive direction. It's time for us to change the topic for now.
- Our life experiences cause us to have a difference of opinion. We don't have to agree.
- I'm willing to share my perspective on this, but I'm not willing to be disparaged.
- Your beliefs are harmful and I do not tolerate this kind of talk.
- I see it differently. Are you open to thinking about it from another point of view?

Your beliefs and how strongly you hold them will determine if you delay a conversation, change the topic altogether, or communicate an intolerance for someone's words. Not every disagreement will end the same way. Consider how your social interaction impacts your emotional well-being. The overlap of your areas of wellness will be discussed more in chapter 5. Intellectual conversations have the potential to energize you cognitively without boundaries. However, if they drain you emotionally, or challenge you spiritually, addressing these in a way that honors the other person's dignity and allows you to be true to you is done by establishing intellectual boundaries. It is wise to maintain an awareness of how a challenging dialogue impacts you and what boundaries will be most helpful to protect.

Material Boundaries

How people access and handle your possessions is another area where having boundaries can communicate how you expect your material items to be treated. Think about what possessions people can use, how they can acquire them, and the care they exhibit when in their custody. Others may not know that the pen on your desk was a gift and a prized possession, one you don't want out of your sight. Or maybe you're happy to share a copy of a good book, but would like it returned without markings or folded pages.

Most often, if you simply tell someone what you are comfortable with and what you are not, they will gladly comply. If you fail to speak your mind, it could be too late and you'll hear something that starts with, "If I had known . . ." The following statements are options for making sure people understand how to use and treat your property.

- You can use my coffee maker anytime, just bring your own pods.
- You are welcome to borrow my car as long as you replace the gas you use.
- I have a speaker you can use any day except Tuesday when I need it for an activity.
- If you borrow a book, please put a sticky note on my desk to let me know you have it.
- You may choose to sit in any of these seats except this one.

Look Up

Your eyes communicate a lot to someone. A glance away from people sends a nonverbal message that you are not inviting interaction. See what happens when you look at people when you're in public places. Make eye contact and offer a "hi" to people you come in contact with. The benefits of reciprocated greetings and smiles can be a lift for both of you. A simple hello can help you connect to people at a more personal level.

Sign Up

If your calendar is not already overcommitted, volunteering at community and school events is an excellent way to connect with others. Offer to help with the football game concession stand; this will surely keep you busy and you will be interacting with many of the other volunteers and community purchasing hot dogs and other snacks. If being around hot dogs and nachos on a cool fall evening isn't your idea of a good time, there is no shortage of community organizations that are in need of people to help with events.

Classify Your Social Media

It's in the title—*social m*edia. Interacting with others online is labeled for socialization. The potential drain social media can have on other areas of your overall wellness must be weighed against the advantages you actually gain by engaging on various platforms. Addictive apps or games coupled with too much exposure to blue light impacts your ability to sleep. The negativity, judgement, and artificial positivity found on many sites leads to low esteem. False information or opinions disguised as fact cause you to be misinformed about potentially critical topics. The disadvantages of social media are plentiful.

However, there are some benefits to connecting online. When social media is used to build your professional learning network, stay connected to loved ones, or plan activities with groups of friends or family, it is a powerful and helpful tool. The problem is, even with the best of intentions, the consequences of the downside of social media are challenging to avoid.

Classify your interactions on social media. Consciously label the purpose for the app or activity. Are you on Twitter to build your professional learning network? Then use the strength you've built through mindfulness to focus solely on the purpose of connecting with other educators who teach your same subject or grade level. Perhaps you're interested in going gradeless. Then follow thought leaders like Starr Sackstein and join conversations she's having with others and continue to grow your network of professional support and growth.

If you find yourself spending hours and hours of Candy Crush every day, consider how that is impacting your social wellness. Likewise, if you intend to hop on Facebook to see what's new with your brother and his family, again, be mindful and get your update and consciously avoid the posts that trigger a withdrawal from other areas of your wellness. The classification of your social media activity will help you differentiate when your time is helpful and when it is a hindrance. The clarity of the labels enables you to choose and manage how social media impacts you.

Grow Your Professional Learning Network (PLN)

A strong social network can be essential to help you through stress. The impact of maintaining positive social relationships is linked to different aspects of health and wellness. This is true in both your personal and professional lives. Professional learning networks support social, cognitive, and emotional aspects of teacher growth (Trust et al., 2016). For many educators, their school or professional network feels like a family.

Teachers often have little choice in who is part of their school family. When challenges arise at school, having a network of other professionals beyond your home community offers an outside perspective on issues you might be facing. Sometimes a third party who understands the intricacies of a situation but does not have the complexity of the personalities involved can provide you with the clarity you need to work through a conundrum.

Professional learning networks are support groups focused on your profession. While they include your school family, strong PLNs include other educators and experts outside your district. Reaching out to people across the country is not as convenient as stopping someone in the hallway, but social media lessens the effort. If you haven't built a PLN beyond your geographic area, look for groups on Facebook, follow a Twitter hashtag like #edchat, or search Pinterest for "brain break" or some other area of interest to find posts, people, and entities that offer suggestions.

If you find yourself going down a rabbit hole searching for kitchen organization tools, pause and determine if the time spent here will benefit your cognitive wellness by decluttering your pantry or if your time on Pinterest is no longer serving your intended purpose of growing your PLN. Then, based on the impact on your overall wellness, start sorting soup cans or log off the social media platform.

Let Others Serve You

The idea of reaching out to others when you're down or need an emotional boost was offered in chapter 2. Circles of close-knit individuals permit you to use this strategy when you need it. Consider explicitly asking someone in your circle if you can call on them when you need something. Then—do it! Do not dismiss the benefits that serving others has on an individual. Allowing someone to provide service to you causes them to feel worthy, helpful, and valued.

There is a caution to be acknowledged. Over-requesting help from those close to you has the potential to cause others to feel used or that their time is not important. Note the frequency and the demands you place on others. You do not want to cause strain and drain for them by asking for help more often for convenience than necessity.

Avoid Toxic Relationships

We have all been around a toxic staff member and it can be an absolutely miserable situation. Toxic people bring negativity to the workplace, which directly affects other colleagues. These toxic people drain your energy, productivity, and happiness. In a study from Georgetown University, 98 percent of people indicated they have experienced toxic behavior at work (Bradberry, 2016; Blanding, 2018). These types of interactions at work negatively influence people; 80 percent of respondents lost time worrying about the incidents and 78 percent reported that their commitment to the organization declined (Bradberry, 2016).

Discover where negativity is triggered for you; These areas could be anywhere, such as the staff lounge, the copy room, or the stands at your child's little league game. When possible, limit your time in the areas that you identify as negative. Best-selling author Robert Sutton advises to stay more than 100 feet from a toxic person, if you are within 25 feet of the person, the chances that you are going to be in a toxic situation increases (Lynch, 2017).

If you must interact with the toxic person, emotionally distance yourself and do not open up to them; be friendly and positive, but stay somewhat removed to avoid being in a situation that brings frustration to you. Use self-care strategies routinely to take care of yourself and stay strong in your positive attitude around toxic colleagues or supervisors.

Get Comfortable with "No"

It can be difficult to say no to something or someone, but it is a skill that educators should embrace and apply when needed. Healthy boundaries, as shared previously in this chapter, are an essential component of self-care. Poor boundaries in our work or personal relationships can lead to resentment, anger, and burnout. For teachers, setting boundaries can help avoid burnout and lead to remaining in the profession longer. Boundaries are decisions we make that govern our behavior and the way we interact with others (Miller & Lambert, 2018). These boundaries can include how we spend our time, our emotional involvement, and our independence and reliance on others.

It is acceptable and productive to set a boundary by saying no. Even though committing to everything you're asked might cause others to see you as dependable and cooperative, it likely causes another area of your wellness to suffer. Saying yes to one person inevitably means saying no to someone or something else. That someone might be YOU. Many times people continue to ask the people who are eager to assist. But, you need to agree to things in moderation, not full force.

Designate "No Screen" Time

Whether you're one-on-one or in a group, be completely present with those you're interacting with. Put your phone in your pocket or on the counter and fully engage with others. One study revealed that Americans check their phones over 250 times per day. That's about every 3 minutes and 48 seconds of your waking hours (Wheelwright, 2021). Eighty-nine percent of people indicated that during their last social interaction, they took out a phone and 82 percent shared that it deteriorated the conversation (Suttie, 2015). As you're building your social wellness, consider how giving your attention to your device makes them feel.

The impact of choosing technology over the human you're with is not diminished with a fleeting "I'm sorry" or an explanation of what you're reading. If someone is sharing a story and you interrupt their story by explaining that your repairman is confirming your appointment for tomorrow, the unintended message remains; you gave less than your full attention to the person in your social circle. Seldom are messages that get our immediate attention time sensitive. Most often, your alerts can wait.

Tag Along

Join a friend, colleague, or family member when they are running errands. This can be an occasion to get some needed items or simply ride along as you spend time with another person. The opportunities to tag along could include various errands or a shopping trip to a mall or store. You may decide to window shop and not purchase anything, but enjoy the moment and time with another person.

Interview a Family Member

Consider who you would like to know more about seek out a conversation to learn about them. There may be quite a bit you don't know about your aunt, or grandparent. Dedicate an afternoon to find out more about this person's life. You may decide to capture this interview in a video and edit it for future viewing. Some teachers encourage their students to interview someone who has firsthand experience with historical events. There is a lot to be learned about the 1960s by speaking to someone who remembers when John F. Kennedy was president. The interest in someone else's life and perspective strengthens important relationships.

Establish Traditions

Celebrate with others. Use your creativity to ignite a meaningful practice. Create traditions such as special birthday parties, a Fourth of July cookout, and holiday celebrations. Summer may be a time that you gather the family camping and playing games, whereas winter time hosts events such as a day of baking goodies for others. These family customs are often passed down between friends and generations. The memories, socialization, and positive feelings formed from these experiences are everlasting.

Have a Date Night

Schedule time on your calendar for a weekly date night. These evenings can be romantic outings with your significant other or events that you both enjoy. Dinners, bowling, visiting a museum, movie night, and attending a concert are some plans that may spark your interest. Include activities throughout the dates that you both enjoy, and share selecting the events, such as rotating who decides on what the destination will be for the night.

Notification List

Select groups of interest and sign up for newsletters about social events planned by these businesses or organizations. You will be able to see up-to-date information on the latest news and invitations. Choose to invest your time in the happenings that are significant to you and spark enthusiasm. Another way to know what events are available is a simple app called Meetup. It organizes online groups and connects new people who share similar interests through online and in-person events. That way you won't miss a fun and new activity in your area.

WHEN YOU NEED A SOCIAL FIX

Alarming numbers of people who report loneliness continue to rise. In 2018, even before the pandemic of 2020, nearly half of U.S. adults reported feeling sometimes or always alone (Dodgson, 2018). In her meta-analytic review, Julianne Holt-Lunstad (2010) likened the impact of lack of social connection to health risks such as smoking 15 cigarettes a day, having an alcohol use disorder, or obesity. She says, "Being connected to others socially is widely considered a fundamental human need—crucial to both well-being and survival."

As previously noted in this chapter, some people are more comfortable being alone than others; they might even rejuvenate when they are solo. However, even these folks require human connection and the feeling of love and belonging that our social groups provide. When you're feeling the urge to break a spell of isolation and experience human bonding, try one of the following strategies to give you the social boost you need to nourish your relationships or provide opportunities to create new ones.

Catch Up with Old Friends

Technology allows convenient ways to reach out to people we might otherwise grow apart from. Send a text, message, or call to someone you miss and catch up. Or, better yet, set up a time to meet up for coffee or invite them over for dinner. If you don't have quick access to their phone number or email, you can send them a direct message on a social media platform such as Facebook, Instagram, or Twitter without reading your feed. Remember, keep your intent in mind so social media does not divert you from your goal of simply touching base.

Hug with Care

Touch is an important sense that allows us to reach out to others by forming and maintaining social relationships. Hugging is calming, creates bonds, increases well-being, and lowers stress. In a study conducted in 2014 of over 400 adults, researchers found that hugging may reduce the chance a person will get sick (Cohen et al., 2015). The participants in the study who had the greatest support systems were among the least likely to get sick or have severe symptoms compared to other participants with little or no support system.

Whether you are giving or receiving a hug, make sure the person getting the hug is alright with the contact. There may be limitations on what someone is comfortable with regarding hugging, so ensure you are aware of your relationship with the person and their stance on hugs.

Link with Society

Check your community's events page to find upcoming activities and commit to attending with someone you would like to bring along. Outdoor concerts, a farmer's market, or a lantern walk on a local hiking trail might be waiting for you and a friend. Local libraries and chambers of commerce sponsor gatherings for the public. Discover what picques your interest and mark it down on your calendar to attend.

Get Your Game On

Play is not only important for children. Adults enjoy games too. Dust off the chessboard and teach your daughter how to play, head to the driving range and hit a bucket of golf balls, or make plans to take your family to an escape room. Games are something that can be enjoyed all year long. The lazy hazy days of summer create an opportunity for outdoor games, while evenings or rainy days elicit board games and puzzles. Winter weather evokes a desire to build a campfire, sip a warm drink, and play games that only involve conversation like "Would You Rather?" Establish a card game night with coworkers or friends such as euchre or crazy eights, and enjoy planning and laughing together.

Schedule Social Time on Your Calendar

Some days you may be able to spontaneously join others, but that is not always feasible in the busy life of an educator. If you're not able to do something last minute, add a social commitment to your calendar to give you something to look forward to. Scheduling activities in advance not only allows you to prepare, but it gives you multiple opportunities to connect with your friend, colleague, or partner as you plan for the big day.

Send a Text to Someone Who Makes You Smile

Offering a "What's new?" or "Thinking of you" message to someone in your contacts is an easy way to let them know they're on your mind and initiates an interaction that might be just what you need to lift your spirits. You can always send just a positive emoji such as a happy face or flower. This only takes a few seconds and can be very impactful for the person on the receiving end. Your effort communicates the value you have in the relationship.

Send Snail Mail

In today's world, so much communication is done electronically. Birthday wishes are sent on social media posts and congratulations are offered with a "like" click. Send a card or note through the United States Postal Service. In a day when most mail deliveries are advertisements and bills, your envelope will surely be noticed and appreciated. The recipient is likely to reach out to you to share their gratitude, initiating another interaction.

Show Up

If people in your circle are not available to hang out with you today, choose a public place where you're likely to see and meet other people. Take your canine to the dog park and talk with other pet owners, head to the golf course and join up with others to make a foursome, go to the makeup counter at the mall and ask for a demo or tutorial, or check to see what time the next gym class begins and work out with others. Find interest groups and clubs that welcome new members; check for community events websites or special Facebook groups in your area.

BELL-TO-BELL CONCENTRATION ON SOCIAL PROSPERITY

Positive relationships with teaching colleagues make the job of teaching more enjoyable. Fostering trust and respect within your school family is valuable because you spend so much time around them. This section focuses on ideas for you to connect with your colleagues on a social level. A blend of personal rapport and professional regard makes for the perfect balance at work.

A sense of humor and a bit of fun between bells seem to make the day go faster and keep the school as a place where you enjoy being. Try some of these ideas or use them to inspire new ways to concentrate on your social relationships, even when you're in the instructional mode.

Buddy-Up

Partner with another classroom to read to younger students or learn something new from more advanced students. Combining classes to work together encourages growth among students, but also allows staff members to foster their relationships. The ideas for potential integrated topics are endless; you may decide to use reading as a connector, a science, technology, engineering, and mathematics (STEM) project, or a service project such as sprucing up the school grounds.

Co-Teach with a Colleague

Combine classes across content. Students enjoy a change in activities, and co-teaching with a fellow teacher is a way to add some variety in teaching and learning. The shared responsibility of two adults creates a bond that enhances collaboration skills. The teacher partnership grows, and students are afforded the opportunity to see a joint effort. Teachers and students are exposed to more people during this process and are able to interact with a variety of skill sets.

Arrive Two Minutes Earlier

Build in time to start your day off with a social connection. Show up to school two minutes earlier than you normally have scheduled and make a point to say hello to another staff member, using those two minutes to intentionally focus on the person in front of you. Start out by arriving two minutes early one day a week, and then work your way up to three days a week as you make the effort to direct your attention to greet a variety of coworkers. Two minutes in the morning is manageable for you and your colleague. Be fully present as you wish them a good morning, and then move on to your classroom so you can center on teaching and learning.

Have a Hallway Hangout

Between classes, as you observe the hallways, find another teacher to chitchat with when you're not connecting with students. These precious minutes can be used to share, laugh, and smile. You have limited time according to the schedule and when class needs to begin, so make your conversation succinct and friendly. This is not the moment to get carried away and lose track of time, but to interact concisely before you return to teaching.

Activate 2x10

Spend 2 minutes with one student for 10 consecutive school days, with a particular student talking about anything the student wants to discuss. This strategy helps build a relationship and rapport with the student. This safe conversation allows students to share personal interests. If the child isn't sharing right away, ask open-ended questions to foster the communication. When you ask follow-up questions like, "How did your visit with your uncle last night?" students will know you were listening and had interest in what they have been sharing with you.

Plan with a Partner

Share brain power and connect with someone in your department or grade level to plan lessons and activities. The collaboration can help reduce the work by consolidating efforts. Working together is working smarter. On days when you are out of the classroom, your partner, who is familiar with what you had planned, can be a valuable resource for your substitute.

Don't Send It

Email is immediate and easy to just send away. If your message is not time sensitive, walk down the hall and have a face-to-face conversation instead. The in-person discussion encourages relationship building and clear communication; sometimes emails can be misinterpreted. In our fast-paced world of emails and messages, a face-to-face interaction is appreciated.

Pair and Ride Share

By riding to work with another person, you are not only saving gas, but you are able to enjoy a coworker's company. It makes sense to take turns driving, but if one person prefers to always drive, contribute some money for gas. Leave your route a few minutes early every Monday to stop and get your favorite morning drink or treat and kick off the week with some extra enjoyment.

GIVE AND GET BACK SOCIALLY

Bringing together people may be an area where you excel and you are more than willing to share your talent. If you're an extrovert, you probably thrive on it. Your understanding of how helpful social interactions are is something you can facilitate and make more accessible to others. This might include planning events, initiating social and emotional support, or creating opportunities for folks to expand their social circles.

Check In/Check Out

Stop to say hello or goodbye to a colleague you know is facing some struggles or doesn't seem to be him/herself lately. A few moments spent with this person can be so meaningful to them. The effort to intentionally find them and give a cheerful greeting doesn't have to continue into a conversation that requires a large chunk of time. The idea of checking on someone is a small way to let them know you care.

Uncover Interesting Facts

Coordinate a fun activity that helps staff members get to know one another better. Staff can bring in their baby photos or kindergarten photos and everyone will need to match the past picture with the current-year school picture. If staff members have pets, they could bring in a pet photo, and others can try to connect the pet with the owner.

Lift 'Em Up

The staff lounge should be a place of comfort and safety. Teachers cannot allow negativity to surround the staff gathering area. As in many situations, it can be easy to complain, but focus on keeping the talk positive. If the talk does stray, help bring it back with these example phrases.

- That has not been my experience.
- I really enjoyed the assembly.
- What source are you using for that information?
- Everyone has their unique experiences.
- How can we help?

Send Invitations

Invite anyone to join you in an activity that benefits them, but in a social atmosphere. Options such as a 15-minute walk around the building or campus after school or joining you for a mindful moment before school begins don't have to take long. If your school is embracing a new initiative or promoting a theme for a set period of time, organize a make-and-take where educators can create resources for bulletin boards, student rewards, or tools for lessons. You might feel comfortable around everyone in the building, and some teachers might feel there are cliques. Send invitations to everyone so a variety of relationships can bloom.

Plan Events

Put a social gathering on the school calendar and invite folks to meet up to unwind. The staff may decide to designate a day and make this a weekly or monthly standing event. The ongoing and open invitation will reduce pressure people might have that they are expected to attend, and provides multiple invitations for them to consider. Time outside the classroom is precious, so if your colleagues choose to spend time with family over meeting up for happy hour, don't be offended. Survey people to get a picture of what could make it more attractive for people to attend. Maybe they're tired by Friday, and swapping a social get-together on a Sunday afternoon at a local coffee shop would be more convenient.

Give the Best Medicine

Laughter is contagious. Share funny stories or events with staff. This might be something hysterical a kindergartener said, or that you just happen to be wearing two different shoes today. Shared laughter strengthens our relationships by communicating to others that we have a similar world view (Suttie, 2017).

FEATURE THE TEACHER WITH SOCIAL WELLNESS

A group of educators from a middle Atlantic state have found a way to stay socially, emotionally, and academically connected with each other. These seven teachers have a private back channel, via group text, they use all year long. One day after an interesting lunch conversation, the educators had an urge to continue discussion on their topic. This is how their group chat was born. Over the years, the name of the group changes based on the current headline they're discussing.

A simple conversation has transcended into what one of the teachers called a "lifeline" for them to stay connected and feel supported. They message one another for just about anything. Examples include questions about novels they're studying with students, parental triumphs, and even heads up that administration is doing walkthroughs. The trust and social connection is built on thousands of interactions over multiple years of working together.

One teacher in the back channel group shared that she communicates with her school group more than she does with some members of her family. The group doesn't limit their messages to school topics either. They've grown to share personal victories and provide empathetic ears in a time when so many educators are burdened with influences that strain them more than necessary.

Their closeness has generated inside jokes that keep them chuckling during difficult times. At the time of publication, the name of their chat group had recently been changed to "The Circle of Negativity of the Island of Lepers." You might look at this title with confusion, but to the seven members of this social support group, it triggers previous conversations with a speck of current reality that allows them to maintain a positive mindset. AKA, inside jokes.

Sadly, the group requested to be anonymous for fear they might be reprimanded for messaging each other during the school day. Perhaps part of the joy of the back channel is its secrecy. Even so, this is a frightening notion. Even if their worries are unfounded, the fact that any doubt at all exists about whether administration approves, let alone encourages teachers to use their social relationships to support them professionally, is a serious concern. One would hope that school leadership would be eager for teachers to create systems of support to comfort them in times of struggle, lift them in times of bleakness, reassure them in times of worry, and inspire them in times of apathy.

The uncertainty of how this group of surviving educators would be perceived reveals the innate fear teachers have of judgement and ridicule. The pressure to be a role model 24/7 does not leave room for adults in the education profession to be their authentic selves. This conflict between what they believe and how they present themselves impacts their spiritual wellness, which is the topic for the next chapter. As educators find healthy ways that offset the strains of teaching, your social connections just might provide you with the strength to effectively cope when you are feeling drained.

EDUCATOR COMMITMENT TO SOCIAL PROSPERITY

Use these end-of-chapter reflection prompts to process what this chapter revealed for you and your social prosperity.

Table 4.1: Social Care Needs Assessment Checkbox

	Never/ Rarely	Occasionally	Frequently/ Always
I consider myself to be a social person.			
I enjoy learning about and connecting to other people.			
I feel overwhelmed when I'm in a group.			
My socializing impacts my ability to get things done.			
My social calendar feels stretched to the maximum.			
I feel like I don't spend enough time with important people in my life.			
I have trouble getting to know new people.			
I enjoy activities that involve others.			
When there is a social event, I want to attend.			
I love to meet new people.			
I have activities outside school that allow me to socialize with others.			
I work better with others than alone.			
I get bored when I am alone.			
I spend more time than I should chitchatting.			
I have difficulty initiating conversation.			
Other people enjoy my company.			
I intentionally tend to my social wellness.			
I can recognize when I need a social boost.			
My social care backpack has strategies that help me in this area of wellness.			

1. How has my definition of social wellness been confirmed or shifted?
2. What new perspectives have I gained about social health?
3. What are some ways I can intentionally build my social well-being?
4. What new ideas or strategies have I acquired?

Now, apply your understanding of social wellness and reflect on your own self-care. Table 4.1 offers some statements to help with a needs assessment. Now that you have your checklist completed, search for patterns in your strengths and areas of need. Use the social meter assessment model found in Figure 4.1 to categorize where you want to work to improve, how you plan to continue what is working, and how you might broaden your success to support others. An equal distribution in the need, maintain, and share sections within your social meter assessment model is unlikely. Don't force yourself to find more evidence if it appears you have uncovered enough information for

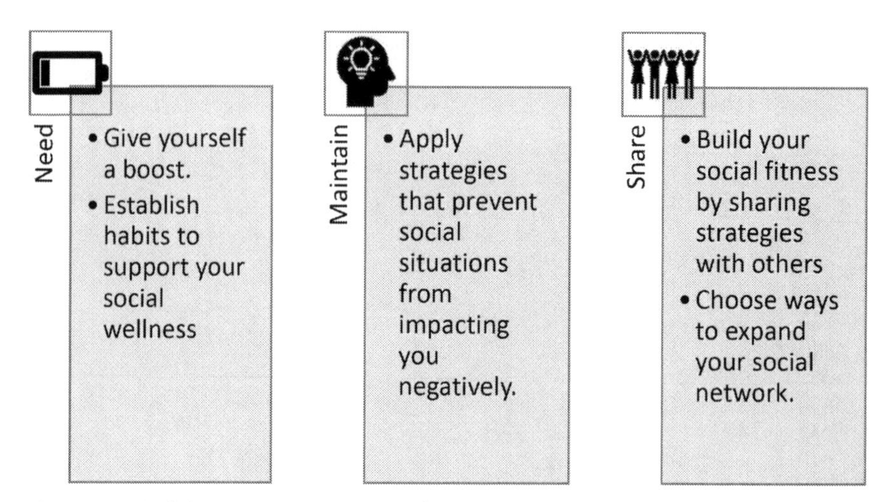

Figure 4.1: Social Meter Assessment Level. ***Source:*** **Connie Hamilton**

you to start a plan. You can always repeat this step and discover new areas to focus your social building attention on.

The areas you identified to address first are directly aligned with sections from this chapter. The examples you placed in the need category will be best addressed by establishing habits that prevent a negative impact on your social health. If your need is temporary or mild, a social boost might be the way to leverage relationships to team socially to address your area of need. Examples of what seems to be working and you desire to continue could be embedded as a routine or mindset that becomes your mantra. Finally, the areas where you thrive and perhaps find personal benefit can be shared with others to contribute to the well-being of those around you. Identify the areas you would like to address first to improve how you address the social aspect of your overall care.

Table 4.2 is where you're going to create your action plan. Walk through the cognitive steps of exploring how areas of your social wellness impact you

Table 4.2: Social Wellness Action Plan

Description of Social Area	Impact on Social Wellness	Strategy to Apply
When there is a social event, I want to attend, but don't always have the time.	I overcommit to responsibilities and don't have time to enjoy social events when I'm invited to join. I feel left out.	Reserve time on my calendar to enjoy social activities. Set a goal for X number of events per month and count them up each week to see if I'm on track. If something gets in the way of scheduled social time, I will either reschedule the social event or use my time boundaries to say "no."

in other ways. Then the tool provides a place for you to identify what suggested strategies from this chapter will fill your social backpack. An example is provided for you to get you started. You can list as many strategies as you'd like, but start with one to three strategies to implement. If you need a cognitive jump start, use these reflection questions:

1. How will you build habits that support your social wellness?
2. What will you do to maintain a healthy social self?
3. When necessary, what are some quick boosts to bump your social needs?
4. How can you care for your social self within the school day?
5. In what ways might you share or model the importance of social well-being with others?

As you feel the benefits of your strategies, revisit the action plan to continuously focus on your social self.

Chapter 5

Focus on Spiritual Strength

What brings meaning and purpose to your life? How do your beliefs and morals guide your everyday living? How often do your actions deviate from your values? Experiencing life according to your ethics, principles, and purpose grounds you into who you are as a person. How you identify, connect, and reflect on what you stand for is how this chapter interfaces with self-care. Specifically, the chapter is about your spiritual wellness.

Spiritual health is possessing a set of morals, principles, values, and beliefs that provide a sense of purpose and meaning in life, and using those principles to guide your actions. Your spiritual health is your core, your innermost self—it refers to where you came from, who you are, and where you are headed to achieve your goals. As Stephen Covey shares, "The spiritual dimension is your center, your commitment to your value system. It draws upon the sources that inspire and uplift you and tie you to timeless truths of humanity" (p. 292). People with strong spiritual health have clarity on what they stand for and are able to live their lives close to those ideologies. When your actions reveal the self you aspire to be, you're tending to your spiritual wellness.

RETHINKING MASLOW'S HIERARCHY

Abraham Maslow's hierarchy of needs is a well-known theory of human motivation. He suggests that certain levels of needs must be achieved before a person moves on to the next level. While Maslow has acknowledged that there can be some exceptions to the idea of a strict sequence of obtaining needs, and there is interconnection, he maintained that some human needs were more foundational than others. The image most commonly associated with Maslow's hierarchy, and whose origin is not known (Kaufman, 2019), is a five-part pyramid as shown in Figure 5.1.

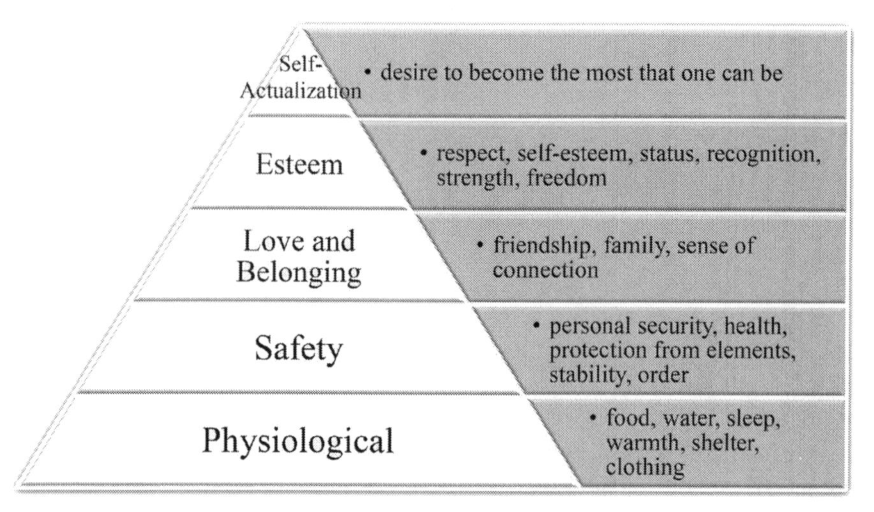

Figure 5.1: Maslow's Hierarchy. *Source:* Created by Connie Hamilton; adapted from info gathered from Maslow A. H. (1969). The farther reaches of human nature. *Journal of Transpersonal Psychology,* 1(1), 1–9.

Physiological needs are at the base of the pyramid followed by safety, love and belonging, and esteem, and self-actualization fills the top. While the pyramid is intended to represent Maslow's original hierarchy, it does not appear to be Maslow's pyramid. Later, Maslow revised his hierarchy into seven sections with transcendence added as the final level (Maslow, 1969).

There is significant evidence that Maslow's hierarchy was inspired by the Siksika (Blackfoot) lifestyle (Blackstock, 2019). It is worth noting that there are some testaments within and outside the Blackfoot tradition that Maslow secured, and then misrepresented their wisdom (Michel, 2014). What is not in question is that Maslow recognized an undeniable difference between the Blackfoot and Western civilization. He noted that "70–80% of the Blackfoot are more secure than the most secure 5% of our population." (Blood & Heavyhead, 2007). Maslow's reflection reveals the cultural bias he brings to his theory. Therefore, when thinking about spiritual wellness, there is much that can be learned by considering varying, even conflicting views from your own. Challenging what you are taught to be true in order to develop your own set of beliefs is part of gaining spiritual clarity.

Terry Cross is the founding director and now senior advisor for the National Indian Child Welfare Association and is a member of the Seneca Nation. He sees Maslow's theory differently. Through indigenous eyes, Cross argues that human needs are interdependent, not hierarchical (Blackstock, 2011). Notice in Figure 5.2 how Cross places spirituality in the center. Teju Ravilochan, cofounder and SEO of the Unreasonable Institute, interprets it

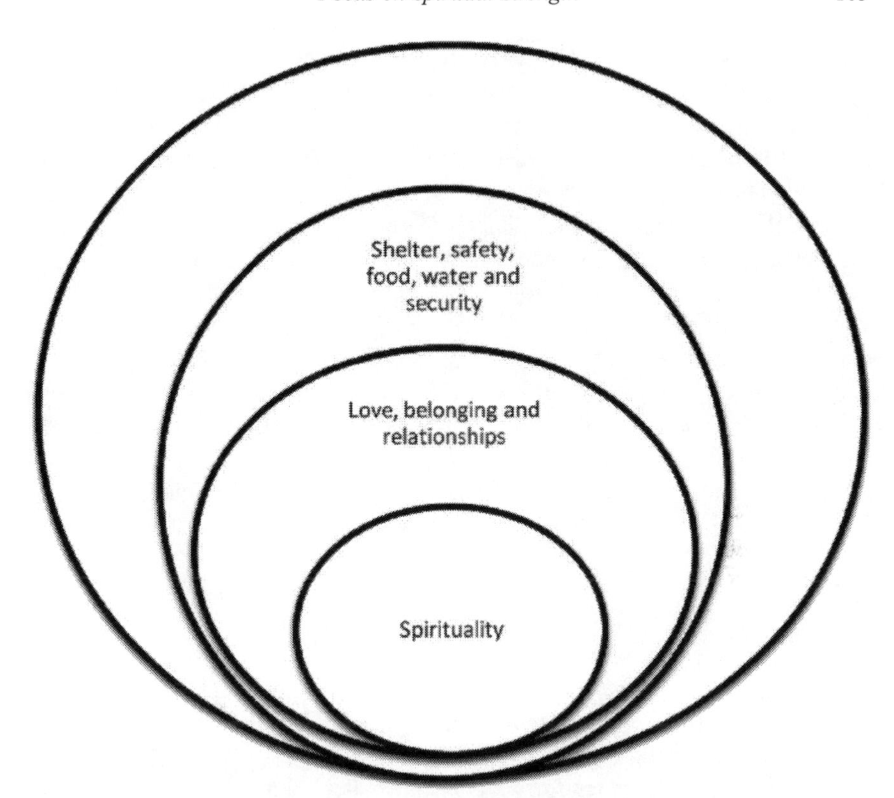

Figure 5.2: Terry Cross's View. ***Source:*** **Blackstock, C. (2011). "The Emergence of the Breath of Life Theory."** ***Journal of Social Work Values and Ethics,*** **8(1).**

this way, "self-actualization is not achieved; it is drawn out of an inherently sacred being who is imbued with a spark of divinity" (Ravilochan, 2021).

Cross's perspective reinforces the importance of having a strong sense of spirituality. Solid examples that bring questions to Maslow's leveling structure are the incidents when individuals sacrifice their own needs for the sake of others. Even the ultimate sacrifice of giving one's life to protect another is innate in many people. Three examples that come to mind include parents willing to suffer so their children don't have to, military willing to die for their country, and countless activists enduring pain and self-sacrifice for causes bigger than themselves. These acts of dismissing basic needs for the purpose of advancing a greater good are, in fact, models of a balance between beliefs and actions, which is at the heart of spirituality.

THE POWER OF PEACE

In order to truly hear their own thoughts, many spiritually sound people commit to listening, processing, and reflecting on their innermost thoughts and feelings. The core of who you are or want to be is what some call your soul; others call it your spirit. In this chapter, we will reference it as your *true self*. Whatever you label it, this chapter is dedicated to helping you get in touch, stay connected, or strengthen your beliefs. Clarity on the principles by which you live is necessary to rely on your true self to make decisions that avoid conflict within yourself.

Moments or even long periods of time when there is a disconnect between behaviors and beliefs lead to contradiction. This mismatch of actions that challenge your moral compass can lead to regret, low esteem, and a wider gap between how you see yourself and how others see you. This is why it is important to nourish your relationship with yourself just as you care for your relationships with loved ones, colleagues, and your students.

Throughout this chapter, there will be a variety of suggestions to grow your spiritual self-care. Discover activities and behaviors that allow you to unearth what is meaningful and to maintain a strong sense of self. Put into practice what works for you within your daily schedule. Spiritual health is a personal journey. Incorporate ideas that are meaningful to you and that are doable within your life's focus.

Because your actions tend to reveal your beliefs and values, you are constantly showing your friends, fellow educators, family, and even strangers your authentic self with every interaction. To help you bring your awareness of spiritual care into focus, respond to the prompts provided, then refer back to them as you read through this chapter.

1. What is my current understanding of spiritual wellness? What do I consider to be my "true self"?
2. How do I tend to my spiritual well-being?
3. In what ways do my actions align or stray from my core values?
4. What is something I hope to learn as I read about spiritual wellness?
5. How would I rate my current spiritual well-being barometer?

LIVING WITH SPIRITUAL COMFORT

There are two key concepts to tending to your spiritual care: First is obtaining clarity on what you want your mantra to be. The second is how well your actions project your mantra to others. The goal is to have a tight alignment where you develop a sense of peace and comfort because your actions support your true self and your true self guides your actions. This reciprocity continuously feeds your spirituality and can bring harmony to your life.

In music, harmony is when multiple chords are played at the same time and produce a pleasant effect. When referencing spiritual care, harmony is the supportive relationship between the core of your being and the interactions you have day to day. When they match, it produces a pleasant feeling that can be described as peace, contentment, joy, fulfillment, or tranquility. Tending to your spiritual self is critical to contentment, but also in creating a strong foundation so when life hands you lemons, you have the strength to cope and continue to move forward in a lemonade of peace.

The Mayo Clinic (Sparks, 2019) reports that spirituality has many benefits for stress relief. COVID was a major curveball for many, and stress levels have multiplied during the COVID-19 pandemic (American Psychological Association, 2021). Educators need to focus on healthy habits by cultivating and creating a sense of purpose, joy, belonging, and sharing. Scientists have discovered repeatedly that those having a spiritual practice tend to be happier than those who don't (Walsh, 2017).

Some people seek to align their lives with their doctrine to experience joy and fulfillment. Core values and pillars are outlined in some religions for their members to follow. While spiritual wellness does not have to be connected to religion, traditions within religions are often ways individuals maintain focus on their true selves. Clearly, being "religious" doesn't automatically make someone spiritually strong. Likewise, people who do not believe in a divine being or higher power are not destined for spiritual weakness.

Religion is undoubtedly a way to tap into your true self, but it doesn't define your level of spiritual wellness. As you continue on your spiritual wellness path, remember that you must center on your values and what brings you solace. Focus your intentions on personal convictions as you are the one who understands your virtue.

Building habits into your life that encourage you to explore your true self and reflect on how you're living will strengthen your spiritual self. Add any suggestions to your spiritual health backpack that help you explore more about this area of your wellness.

Mindfulness

The education profession requires teachers to juggle multiple thoughts at a time. During a lesson, teachers are managing learning purpose, time, attending to non-verbal cues from students, analyzing the success of the lesson, assessing understanding of the concept or skill, determining how to adjust instruction or tasks in the moment, measuring engagement, and more. This doesn't even speak to the external thoughts that creep into teachers' minds that are not related to the lesson. Am I prepared for the IEP after school today? Will I have time to call a parent? Don't forget to share sign-up sheets for tutoring. When can I find a moment to speak to a student privately? Added to these thoughts and wonderings are things related to life outside school such as family, and other areas of your self-care like food and warmth.

If you live in this constant state of managing multiple thoughts, it makes it challenging to give 100 percent of your attention and energy to any single one. This is exactly what mindfulness combats. The purpose of mindfulness is to be present in the moment and to focus on the here and now. Therefore, bringing mindfulness into your life can help you give your full attention to the areas you want to focus on and bring your attention inward.

With so many influencers around you, it's easy for your inner voice to be lost in the noise of society, media, and the opinions of others. Quieting those influences, even for a moment, gives a voice to your true self. When your inner voice grabs hold of the microphone, it's easier to listen to yourself, to determine if thoughts or words from others complement or conflict with your own pillars.

People spend approximately 47 percent of their time thinking about something other than what they are doing, and these wandering thoughts are leading to unhappiness (Killingsworth & Gilbert, 2010). It is time to calm the busyness in the mind and listen to your own intuition. People who practice mindfulness tend to have less anxiety, greater empathy, and compassion. Utilizing mindfulness alleviates stress, which can lead to a better mood and better ability to handle stress (Remmers et al., 2016).

Having the mental control to bring forth thoughts and, perhaps more importantly, to let go of distracting thoughts is an essential skill to moving toward a peaceful state. When you think of calmness, you likely imagine minimal areas of focus. The ability to be mentally aware and have influence over your thoughts is necessary to intentionally reflect on anything.

Teachers who are strained and drained often experience unhealthy levels of stress because they have too many important things to manage. The attempt to solve one problem or focus on one need is often interrupted by more problems and needs. This vicious cycle is one factor that increases stress.

Mindfulness helps people construct a buffer between their jobs and becoming burned out in their work (Taylor & Millear, 2016). Do you ever get mesmerized by patterns or lost in a song? These are examples of ways your brain is holding on to a single thought or event. When you bring mindfulness into your routine, it means you don't wait for these moments to occur. Instead, you purposefully dedicate time to practicing the skill of quieting everything except a single focal point. You then hold that focus for as long as you can. This exercise strengthens your ability to isolate thoughts when you need to because you have increased your mind's ability to set a target and keep it in your sights.

The ability to have that level of attentiveness whenever you want or need it is beneficial to your spiritual care. When it's time to get in tune with your true self, you will be better able to make that connection and hold it for long enough to explore your thoughts. This quiet exploration can bring clarity to decisions you need to make, feelings you have about events in your life, or offer self-guidance on how to be the best version of you.

Take Ocean Breaths

Ocean breathing, also known as Ujjayi, is a breathing tool that combines deep breathing with the sound of the ocean to create focus, calm, and clarity. This technique allows you to quiet the mind and listen specifically to your inner voice. When using Ujjayi, inhalation and exhalation are done through the nose. The gentle pulling the breath in and gently pushing the breath out creates a soothing sound, like the sound of ocean waves moving in and out.

Smell the Goodness

Scents can bring back memories and affect mood and feelings. Some people find significant value and comfort in smells, which allows them to center on the aroma and elicit a sense of peace. Aromatherapy can heighten your senses and stimulate the receptors in your nose, which sends messages through the nervous system to your brain.

Aromatherapy uses essential oils that are derived from plants. Fragrant essences and incense, such as balsam and frankincense, have been used throughout history in spiritual tales and traditions. Lavender is a popular scent for relaxing and calming. There are a variety of ways to utilize essential oils, some include simply smelling, placing on the skin, and pouring in a bath. Diffusers distribute the scent without placing the oils directly on your skin. Select the scents that evoke the most pleasant experiences for you.

Daily Mindful Moments

Nourish your mindset to set aside the hustle and guide your thoughts to your innermost devotion. Dr. Amit Sood, the chair of the Mayo Mind Body Initiative, shared a way to assist in the daily practice of mindfulness (Campbell, 2015). He suggested gratitude, compassion, acceptance, meaning, and forgiveness as areas of focus. His advice was to isolate a single virtue for each day's practice to give it your full attention. Use the suggestions provided to guide you through mindful moments each school day.

Monday Gratitude

Recognize and be thankful for things in your life. Gratitude has been referenced throughout the book. That's because it has benefits that span multiple areas of your self-care. As it relates to your spiritual wellness, gratitude serves to anchor you. It calls to mind what you appreciate and keeps your priorities in focus. Your priorities are directly connected with your true self, so acknowledging them feeds positivity to your spirit. When taking your gratitude inventory, be sure to include not only the opportunities you have but also the obstacles you do not have.

Tuesday Compassion

Acknowledge the frustration of others and do something to help lessen it. Compassion goes a step beyond simply caring for someone else. It requires you to take action and show your kindness. Empathy and compassion go hand in hand. The extension of compassion offers grace for imperfections and efforts to diminish pain or suffering someone else might endure.

Wednesday Acceptance

For educators who are modest, accepting gifts, including compliments, is not easy. People who do not like to be the focus of attention tend to dismiss recognition, especially praise. The root causes for difficulty receiving accolades vary. It could be the receiver is a perfectionist, has a negative image of themself, or is afraid of being viewed as egotistical. Depending on the relationship between the giver and the receiver, an underlying assumption of doubt around the authenticity of the compliment might exist. In this case, the risk of accepting a hollow sentiment could lead to humiliation for believing it was delivered as a truth.

When someone offers you a gift, whether it's a physical present or comes in the form of a verbal offering, respond with a "thank you." Resist the urge to undercut your worthiness of the praise or gift. Also, reciprocating the compliment with an equaled praise phrase such as "you, too" devalues the affirmation given to you. By turning the focus back on to the receiver, you fail to acknowledge the compliment bestowed upon you.

On the other end of the spectrum of acceptance is knowing what is in your control and what is out of your control. In the circumstances when you're handed a bucket of sh!t, your spiritual self will suffer if you perseverate on how crappy life is. A healthier view is to mindfully choose how you want to address it. As discussed in chapter 2, you have four options: solve the problem, feel better about the problem, tolerate the problem, or stay miserable. When you practice acceptance, you are essentially helping yourself to feel better about the problem. In turn, you will be able to leave your bucket behind and carry on with your life in a healthier spiritual way.

Thursday Meaning

This is the heart of your spiritual wellness. In this case, meaning is not a link to your cognitive needs. The reference to meaning in the context of mindfulness is to understand your purpose in life and your contribution to the world. For centuries, philosophers have explored the famous question, "What is the meaning of life?" Your mindful moment should include the personal perspective on this question. What meaning does *your* life have? To create a spiritual balance, live your life in a way that makes your answer true.

Consider what contributions you provide to the earth and humanity. If you define one of your life's purposes to be to advocating for those who cannot, or do not advocate for themselves, then how are you standing up to wrongdoings when you notice them? If you let them go to avoid conflict, the balance between what you stand for, or your personal meaning, is misaligned with your actions. The disconnection is harmful for your true self.

Friday Forgiveness

Forgiveness is the cure for resentment. It allows you to move on from something that might have caused you harm. Resentment is a common emotion and it can be toxic for the person feeling it. When resentment lingers, it mostly harms the person feeling the negativity. The ability to forgive harm done to you is not a gift for the person who caused the harm. Forgiveness is for you. To forgive is to let go of your anger and resentment so you can move to a better emotional state.

Forgiveness is distinctly different from approval. It's possible to forgive someone without sending the message that the actions are acceptable. Keep in mind that forgiveness doesn't solely apply to others. There may be mistakes you've made in your life that you regret. Regret is like resentment of yourself. You can be freed from feelings of regret if you can find the self-compassion to forgive yourself.

Traumatic events in a person's life often prevent forgiveness from occurring. Unfortunately, it prolongs the pain and suffering the victim feels. If you're struggling with forgiveness, either with someone in your life or yourself, a licensed professional can help you identify the root of your resentment or regret and move toward forgiveness.

Meditation

Meditation is a self-care practice of focused concentration and encourages a healthy sense of perspective and awareness. Meditation improves self-awareness and builds mindfulness. If you are committed to meditate, it is best to set aside a time or put it on your calendar and treat it as a meeting or appointment you cannot miss. Building meditation into your daily routine will help you form a habit of slowing down and offering attention to the things that matter to you.

If you're wondering, "Wherever will I find the time to meditate?" consider how this fixed mindset is preventing you from making your spiritual self-care a priority. Moments can be found by cutting your time on social media by a few minutes, watching a few less videos on YouTube or TikTok, or getting up when your alarm goes off instead of hitting snooze.

Think about your meditation time as a way to prime your true self for the day or reflect on how your actions aligned with your inner mantra at night. Wherever you choose to embed this spiritual habit, it will be powerful to start with just a few minutes at a certain time of day, then slowly increase the time. If you prefer to be guided through your meditation, there are apps like Headspace, Calm, or Insight Timer available that vary in topic and length to fit your preferences.

Label Your Legacy

Living your life in a way that exemplifies what you stand for can only be done if you have done the soul searching and gained clarity on the traits that you wish others to see. How do you want to be remembered? When others think about what you represent, what do you want them to say? Assigning words to what you want your legacy to be makes it easier to make choices to support it. There is a guide at the end of this chapter to help you label your legacy.

If you want to be thought of as a person who is understanding, then empathy, listening, and being slow to judgment are likely behaviors you will need to express consistently. Consistently is the key word. Your legacy can only be true if it defines the way you regularly live your life. If you're occasionally understanding, it might not be an attribute that others use to describe you.

Write It Out in a Gratitude Journal

What are you grateful for that allows you to live your true self? A gratitude journal is a place to freely write and record the good things in life. Journaling provides an opportunity for you to discover a new perspective on what is important and transparency on what you appreciate in life.

Your gratitude journal will help you hone in on your authentic voice, appreciate life's experiences, and reinforce clarity on what is critical as you focus on living a fulfilled life. Designate a time each day to write in your journal, and keep your journal in the same location for consistency in creating a habit. Write for 5–15 minutes each day on things you are grateful for that day; this allows you to express gratitude and develop harmony with your inner self and a larger world.

Wear His Moccasins

A poem written in 1895 by Mary Torrans Lathrap suggests not to criticize others without having a full understanding of their experiences. You might not recognize the poem by its title, *Judge Softly,* but are likely familiar with the line that suggests you "walk a mile in his moccasins." Her stanzas suggest that without a full understanding of someone else's experiences, you couldn't know how you would respond. This famous poetic quote has been used to encourage empathy and compassion for over a century. When you find yourself being harsh with someone else, recall Lathrap's admonition and consider that there might be a load they are bearing that you are not aware of.

Go Big

The benefits of community service have been highlighted in previous chapters. When it comes to spiritual wellness, your service in the form of volunteering will undoubtedly warm your soul. Going big is a related idea, but is a deeper commitment than spending an afternoon cleaning up a mile stretch of highway.

Spiritual wellness means you contribute to something bigger than yourself. Generosity doesn't have to come in the form of financial gifts. Your time, talents, and attention are also forms of contributing to humanity and the world. To go big, in a spiritual way, you are educating, advocating, and actively seeking to make a positive change in our world. Teachers, by nature of the profession, contribute to society through the education of students. Consider what role you might play in improving the education experience for students, if that's how you are inspired to commit to something bigger. If you have a passion for suitable housing for everyone, in what ways are you feeding your passion to know your actions benefit a greater good?

WHEN YOU NEED A SPIRITUAL LIFT

There are predicaments you might find yourself in that feel like a lose-lose. Educators are often faced with difficult decisions about how they allocate their time, for example. You cannot be in two places at once even if you want to accept an invitation from a student to watch him perform in the evening performance of the school play. If the night of the play happens to fall on the night of the week you typically bring dinner to your grandmother—and you canceled on her the last two weeks in a row—you're likely to feel a spiritual dip.

There are also times you may feel unbalanced and sense you need a boost. This might be caused when you feel uneasy about a gray area you're loitering in. Soul searching occurs when you're uncomfortable with something in your life that doesn't fully support your beliefs or align with your values. The trepidation you feel when your morals are challenged, but not completely violated, will often send you into thought and reflection. The goal is to stay true to yourself, square up with what you believe, and respond in ways that leave no question about where you draw a line.

The strategies offered in this section are intended to help you center yourself on your values and make peace with your decisions.

Repurpose Your Calendar

Calendars come in all sorts of themes. There are 365 days of shoes, daily jokes, and even a year of goats. In addition to these crazy examples, there are also calendars that offer daily inspiration, positive affirmations, motivational quotes, religious messages, recovery quotes, and more. Consider investing in a motivational calendar that aligns with your true self. It doesn't even have to be the current year. Pick one up on clearance midway through the year and just use it for the messaging. Choose a 365-day single page type calendar. Rip off the pages that really speak to you and save them for when you need a spiritual boost. You will be able to get more than twelve months' worth of spiritual lift.

Go Back and Reread

In nearly every chapter, the benefits of how journaling supports various areas of your wellness have been shared. Food logs, mood trackers, gratitude notebooks, professional reflection are all ways journaling can serve as a helpful tool. To put your beliefs in the center of your mind, go back and review writings you have poured onto pages that exemplify what you stand for. It might mean revisiting some hard lessons you narrated to avoid repeating them. In the previous section, "Label Your Legacy" was a strategy for making a habit out of your spiritual well-being. If you have labels for your legacy, revisit them when you need a reminder of what is important to you.

Connecting Mind Body and Spirit

Much like meditation encourages a focal point for your thinking, yoga promotes intentionality, focuses on relaxation, and strengthens your ability to control your breathing. All of these benefits support you spiritually by calming you through slow and intentional movements to lower blood pressure and reduce stress. With relaxation comes clarity. As you sort through the many issues or dilemmas you might be facing, approaching them with a clear mind will help you determine what to do.

If you're a yoga rookie or think of yoga solely as a form of contortion, try loading a relaxation yoga routine from YouTube and follow along. You will be surprised by how tension in your muscles is released and how comfortable you feel in your relaxed state.

Keep the Faith

There is a distinction between spirituality and religion. Religion is a community of people who share common beliefs. According to Pew Research Center's American Trends Panel (2021), 72 percent of Americans are affiliated with a religion. These individuals might find their religion to be a source of spiritual strength.

Connecting with people within a religious community can affirm individual beliefs, which is spirituality. Leaders in a faith can offer guidance when a member is faced with moral challenges. Rituals provide structure and time to reflect on the beliefs of the community and how they are absorbed. The teachings on which a religion is based are lessons and can serve as guidance in the lives of its followers. As mentioned at the beginning of the chapter, spirituality exists within religion, but religion is not required for an individual to be spiritually strong.

Hear the Silence

Being still and quiet creates moments to tap into our inner self. This time allows you to dive deeper into your belief system. Your senses deliver messages to your brain constantly. Noise keeps your brain busy listening and interpreting the sounds. By removing auditory distractions, you reduce the information received. Now you have additional energy to focus on yourself.

If a situation causes you stress, silence helps you feel calm and tranquil (Iberlin, 2017). You can listen to your own voice when the sounds around you are quieted.

In life's busyness, finding a quiet spot might not be as easy as it sounds. If you can't obtain actual silence, try drowning out other sounds by playing non-lyrical music, turning on a white noise app, or just spending a few minutes in the laundry room where the bustle of your home stays on the other side of the door, even if it's just a few minutes.

Visit Your Serenity Space

A small childhood cabin, a treehouse in the woods, an abundant flower garden are all examples of places that may offer comfort and solace. Each person has their own experiences and vision of the desired state for peace. Think of a place that brings you comfort, visit this place, and plan to just be comfortable and to sit still to enjoy the surroundings.

Walking the Mindful Path

Integrate awareness of your inner guide and strengthen your ability to focus on the present by incorporating mindful walking into your day. Select a somewhat quiet place to practice and choose a flat path of approximately 15 feet. Stand still at the end of your path, taking time to notice how you feel.

Maintain awareness of each step and the sensation of the movement of your feet and legs. Pay attention to the changes in your feet and your muscles as you move and make contact with the ground. Notice the sounds, smells, and sights. If your mind wanders, keep your thoughts on simply walking to assure you are concentrating on your true self. As you reach the end of your walking path, stand still again and notice the body in a state of ease. Turn around and center on your awareness, and take a moment before walking the path once again.

BELL-TO-BELL FOCUS ON SPIRITUAL STRENGTH

Of all the areas of wellness, spiritual care is the most authentic to who you are as an individual. Educators hold many roles including teacher, friend, romantic partner, parent, sibling, andcolleague. Your ability to stay true to who you are extends to every aspect of your life. If you want to be thought of as a compassionate person, you must display kindness and tenderness. If your definition of self includes generosity, your actions should often include acts of giving and largesse. By nature of the profession, educators are connected to a sense of contributing to the greater good. Sometimes at their own expense. The following strategies describe how educators can tend to their spiritual wellness during the hours of the day they most often put their own needs aside.

Share Mindful Moments

Once you have established your own routine of mindfulness, there are opportunities for you to bring it into your classroom. Students benefit from the process of clearing their minds too. Many students suffer from difficulty staying focused. Introducing students to mindfulness gives them tools to dismiss mental distractions.

There are books and websites designed specifically for helping with mindfulness. Fablefy (https://www.fablefy.com/) is a site focused on using the power of storytelling to integrate mindfulness for students. The Collaborative for Academic, Social, and Emotional Learning (https://casel.org) has numerous resources for teachers to use with students and has connected mindfulness to two core social-emotional skills: self-regulation and self-awareness.

Jar It Up

Anxiety causes worries to spiral in your mind and, oftentimes, they grow. If you find yourself unable to focus on teaching because school-related worries are getting in the way, try a worry jar or notebook. The kinesthetic act of writing down your concern and putting it in a jar or closing your notebook provides the sensation of letting them go. There may be some things you do need to tend to, so permit yourself to review the worries in your jar or reread the worries in your notebook. When you come across a worry that has been resolved, remove it from the jar or cross it off your worry list.

Leave Private Messages

Place a visual reminder of affirmations somewhere in your desk, bag, or a place that is private to you. Some examples of phrases you may want to use to focus on your spiritual health are:

- My every experience is filled with grace and joy.
- I am loving and kind.
- My goals and beliefs are in alignment.
- I am enough each and every day.
- I am valued by many.
- I am unique and that is a good thing.

- I care about my school, community, and the world.
- I am resilient.

Pray Might be a Way

Prayer is a ritual that grounds many in their spiritual beings. There is a wide range of devotional acts in spiritual traditions. It only makes sense to select the form of prayer that embodies your purpose and meaning in life. Quietly repeat a prayer or phrase from a prayer while breathing intentionally. If the idea of prayer is intriguing, find private time during lunch, planning, or before or after work.

Funnel Your Mantra

When you have labeled your legacy, choose one belief that is true to you and secretly target a single student or colleague as a recipient of your kindness. If you identify encouraging others as a keystone of how you live your life, go out of your way to be a cheerleader for your selected beneficiary. You can change the trait you want to exhibit or change the lucky person you intend to dedicate your attention to.

Slow Down

Sometimes you can feel yourself getting worked up about something. When this happens, pay attention to your breathing to determine if you need to slow it down. Deep, slow, long breaths can help calm the situation down for you. Discard the frustration that entered your mind and breathe in positive energy.

Activate a Helping Hand

Find a community need and fulfill it with your students. Service learning projects help students identify ways they can support the community while learning. What better way to practice adding and subtracting decimals than to shop for items to donate to your local food pantry? Since a key component of spirituality is connecting beyond yourself, these types of activities will not only benefit your own heart, they will instill some spiritual care in your students too. Some ideas to get you started:

- Make cards or artwork for a local nursing home and spend time with the residents.
- Clean up the school grounds, district office grounds, or a nearby park.
- Assist at a local donation center in packing and organizing items.

- Coordinate a local blood drive.
- Send cards and care packages to overseas military members.
- Make and give blankets to the homeless shelter.

Get Outta There

Time spent outdoors can connect you to nature and provide a harmonious experience. Time in nature leads to a decrease in anxiety and rumination (Bratman et al, 2015). A good rule of thumb is to get outside in nature about 20 minutes a day. Research indicates spending at least 120 minutes in nature is associated with good health and well-being.

Depending on the weather and location of your school, you may be able to take advantage of trails to go on with students, use an outdoor area for a curriculum lesson, incorporate a field trip that is outside such as a nature center, farm, or zoo. If weather permits, starting an outdoor garden with students could prove rewarding. You could encourage a teaching colleague to combine classes and coordinate an outdoor activity together.

SPRINKLE SPIRITUAL HARMONY

If spiritual care is an area where you thrive, you already have a keen awareness of what you stand for and your actions show your true self. Dig into your spiritual backpack to discover what you are equipped to share. You might recognize that others are not so in tune with their inner self, or the way they handle themselves might cause others to question their morals or personal beliefs. Your experience and confidence can help those around you to follow your lead in living a fulfilled life.

Look for ways you can be a model or support to others who are either not in touch with their core beliefs or have drifted away for some reason. This section will provide you with some ideas to help you find opportunities to share your strength in spiritual wellness.

Bottle It Up

Shower a friend, family member, or coworker with a jar full of goodness. Share your favorite verses or inspirational quotes by writing them on small pieces of paper and placing them in a jar. As you write the messages, you will be reminded of your treasured passages. Decorate the jar if you wish and give the gift of your meaningful messages to others.

Share the Word

Sometimes a book or article offers a cherished perspective that resonates with its reader. If there is a title that provides this for you, pass it along to someone who might appreciate it. You can choose to loan your copy or give a new copy with a personal note of encouragement or explanation about how it was impactful to you.

Extend an Invitation

Inviting another person to join you in activities that feed your spiritual wellness is one way to introduce others to opportunities to care for themselves. An invitation to attend an event that gives you a spiritual lift could serve as a way to share an enlightening experience. Some ideas are a religious service or activity, a hot yoga class, a guided imagery workshop, or a poetry reading at a coffee house.

Pair Up and Connect

The digital world offers a plethora of options to guide people on their paths to spiritual wellness. If there is an app, website, social group, or another tech avenue that seems a good match for someone in your circle, make the suggestion. Then, as an added layer of support, join them on their journey to venture out and try new things.

For example, the app Headspace has articles, meditation exercises, and videos. It also has an option to add "buddies" under the "More" section. Within the app, you and a buddy can meditate at the same time or at different times. You can even track each other's Headspace progress, monitor each other's journey, and give supporting nudges and encouragement.

Share Your Care

Speak gentle words of kindness. Consider expressing your feelings of care for meaningful relationships with others in your life. You may choose to tell your circle of support how grateful you are that they are in your life. You may decide to use different words to show your feelings, but don't miss an opportunity to share your appreciation. The verbal acknowledgment deepens your connection with your circle.

Isolate the Behavior

There are inevitably going to be times when someone's words or actions are hurtful to you. It's tempting to label a person as ungrateful, rude, or selfish. However, consider the possibility that the other person might be experiencing a weak moment or doesn't have a strong sense of their true self.

By presuming a more positive presupposition, you can gently offer a redirection and some grace. For example, if a teaching partner makes a snarky comment, you might want to lash back with the same tone. However, if you define yourself as a forgiving or understanding person, you can be true to yourself and offer the opportunity for your partner to do the same.

Approach a conversation from a space of care and concern. Consider responses that follow a format like, "You don't seem to be your normal self, usually you're (understanding, generous, supportive, upbeat, etc.). Is everything okay with you?" This message communicates that overall you see her as exuding a positive trait and right now, her words are not aligning with that descriptor. One action doesn't define a person, so separating the behavior from the individual maintains honor and regard for them.

Pay It Forward

Your inner voice is guiding your actions. Let the light inside of you shine while you serve the greater good. As you inspire others in connecting to their true self, encourage your friends or family to volunteer with you to spread acts of goodwill. There are a variety of organizations that need support. Reach out to pantries, shelters, places of worship, community organizations, or pet shelters. You will be modeling service to the community while deepening relationships with your family, friends, and colleagues.

FEATURE THE TEACHER WITH SPIRITUAL WELLNESS

Ms. Rachel Niewiada, a middle school choir director in Grandville, Michigan, wakes up each morning and purposefully pinpoints one positive thing that awaits her. As an educator who is in touch with her spiritual self, Rachel wants her students to feel her joy through the way she interacts with them daily. She understands that the energy she brings to school will be mirrored by her students. This will impact the culture of her classroom and spread as her students interact with others throughout the day.

Like anyone, Rachel doesn't always feel chipper and upbeat. Rather than roll the dice to see what type of day it will be, she has developed habits that prepare her to meet the day with positivity. With a sense of gratitude and at least one thing to look forward to in her sights, she takes time on her morning commute to pray, which gives her the focus she needs to maintain optimism when unexpected disappointments come her way.

She practices gratitude and pauses to find joy in even the smallest things. It is not uncommon for Rachel to narrate these noticings in the classroom. She might comment on the beautiful sunshine or relish the flavor of her morning tea. These simple pleasures are part of her mantra to be grateful for life's gifts. As she verbalizes them, her words and actions align with her true self, displaying a strong sense of spirituality.

To maintain this inner strength, Rachel meditates and has also shared guided meditation with her students. Young adolescents often lack emotional control and do not always think before they act in a challenging situation. Empowering them with a tool like mediation helps them slow and calm down then brings them to a state of mind when they can be conscious of what is happening and how they choose to respond. This increases the likelihood they will be thoughtful in their reactions and sets them up for more favorable outcomes.

Students who have learned meditation in Rachel's class can use it whenever they feel they need to take hold of their emotions, connect with themselves, or make decisions that expose the best version of themselves. The ability to control breathing, which is part of her three-minute meditation sessions, is a powerful skill in itself that her students are developing.

Rachel is aware of how keeping her body and mind healthy keeps her centered and able to live her life with brightness. She strives to not only offer the joy of music to her choir students but also show them the joys that can be found every day.

EDUCATOR COMMITMENT TO SPIRITUAL STRENGTH

As you move forward with building spiritual fitness, take time to process what you have learned with the questions listed here. Consider your strengths in the area of spiritual self-care and your growth edges.

1. How has my definition of spiritual wellness been confirmed or shifted?
2. Are my actions aligned with my core values?
3. What are some ways I can expand in the area of spiritual well-being?
4. What new learning have I acquired?

Now, apply your understanding of spiritual wellness and reflect on your own self-care. Table 5.1 show some reflection statements to help with a needs assessment.

Table 5.1: Spiritual Care Needs Assessment

	Never/ Rarely	Occasionally	Frequently/ Always
I have clearly articulated beliefs.			
My life has balance.			
I participate in a spiritual community.			
I take time to meditate.			
My spirit enhances my day.			
I am at peace with my decisions.			
I allow for reflection.			
I feel like I belong.			
I contribute to a cause in which I believe.			
I make a difference.			
My impact on the world is meaningful.			
I listen to my soul to guide me.			
I make decisions with a higher purpose in mind.			
My actions communicate my beliefs.			
My spiritual wellness is important to me.			
I intentionally tend to my spiritual wellness.			
I can recognize when I need a spiritual lift.			
I have skills to tend to my spiritual needs.			
My spiritual care backpack has strategies that help me in this area of wellness.			

In her book, *Dare to Lead*, Brené Brown (2018) shares a comprehensive list of well over 100 words to represent values. The list in Figure 5.3 was inspired by Brown's list and includes other words that you might connect with when articulating your legacy.

Use the following process to narrow down your legacy labels.

1. Go through the list quickly and circle every word that resonates with you.
2. Prioritize the words by taking the number of words you have circled and cross out half of them.
3. Repeat step 2 until you narrow your legacy words down to just a few.

Keep your legacy labels in mind and examine the checklist you completed in table 5.1. Look for areas that do not support your legacy words, actions that make them come to life, and opportunities to share your spiritual strengths. Prioritize areas of your spiritual wellness that will be most impactful.

Think about what actions would promote your spirituality through routines and daily behaviors. Then make your commitment to develop these choices as habits. To avoid depleting one area of your wellness to fuel another, be aware of what is key to the success you have, then make note of what you

Accepting	Cooperative	Friendly	Just	Respectable
Accountable	Courageous	Fun	Kind	Secure
Authentic	Curious	Generous	Knowledgeable	Simplistic
Ambitious	Dependable	Gracious	Loving	Spiritual
Adventurous	Dignified	Harmonious	Loyal	Successful
Balanced	Disciplined	Honest	Open	Tender
Caring	Efficient	Hopeful	Optimistic	Thoughtful
Committed	Equitable	Humble	Patient	Trusting
Collaborative	Ethical	Inclusive	Patriotic	Trustworthy
Compassionate	Fair	Independent	Peaceful	Understanding
Competent	Faithful	Impactful	Powerful	Virtuous
Confident	Forgiving	Insightful	Reliable	Visionary
Content	Free	Joyful	Resourceful	Wise

Figure 5.3: Legacy Labels. *Source:* Created by Dorothy VanderJagt; adapted from Brown, B. (2018). *Dare to lead: Brave work, tough conversations, whole hearts.* Vermilion.

need to continue to maintain the positive results your efforts provide. Figure 5.4 offers guidance on your next steps to address needs, and maintain and share your spirituality.

Spirituality is arguably the center point of your overall wellness. Yet, it feels like it gets the least amount of attention. People generally feel comfortable discussing their strengths and deficits in the physical, cognitive, and social areas of their wellness, and more awareness is being brought to the importance of emotional self-care. However, it isn't often that spiritual wellness is directly addressed. As you are mindful about your contribution to a bigger part of humanity, the following reflection questions might offer valuable meditation or journaling topics.

1. What does my life feel like when it is in balance?
2. How do I define my true self?
3. What larger entity am I a part of in this life?
4. What does peace mean to me?
5. What is my purpose in life?
6. How are my values reflected in my life?

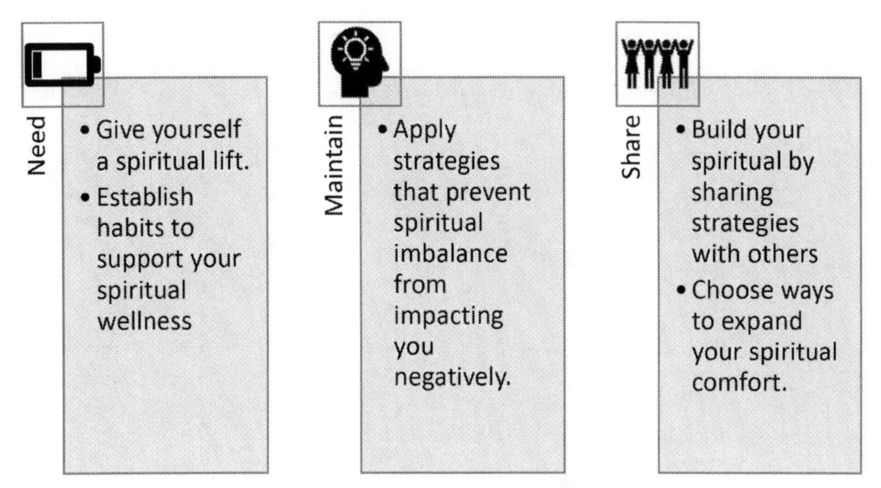

Figure 5.4: Spiritual Meter Assessment Level. *Source:* Connie Hamilton

7. How would others describe my beliefs?
8. If this was my last day, would I be happy with my life?
9. How does my spirituality contribute to my overall wellness backpack?

Chapter 6

Wellness for the Whole Teacher

Now that the compartments of your wellness backpack are filled with actions, you can tend to your personal self-care on a journey to a life of wellness. Physical, emotional, cognitive, social, and spiritual wellness are parts of you as a whole teacher. As you read the first five chapters, you likely saw overlap between the wellness categories shared. This interconnection is something you should be conscious of. The benefits of tending to multiple areas of your wellness in a single event or activity hold great potential for efficiency and balance. However, be cautious of the push and pull relationship they also have. In an effort to tend to one area of need, there is a real risk that you will unintentionally be depleting another.

MULTIPLICATIVE WELLNESS

Multitasking is a myth. Your brain is not capable of performing two cognitive tasks simultaneously. We have the perception of multitasking when we attempt to focus on two tasks at once but what's happening in our mind is that your cognitive energy is quickly switching back and forth over and over. It's like standing up and sitting down; you just can't do them at the same time. Giving the illusion that you are sitting and standing with a blur of up and down movement would tire your thigh muscles in a hurry. The same is true for exhausting your brain when trying to multitask.

If you're not able to do more than one thing at a time, how will you ever be able to juggle five areas of wellness with quality self-care actions? The solution is to reap multiple benefits from single events. Since your wellness is holistic, it's almost harder *not* to double- or triple-dip. For example, what type of self-care would you be using if you were having a healthy lunch with a friend? Physical, because you're nourishing your body? Or you might think social, because you're engaging with someone in your circle. It's both.

One event—having lunch—can be good for you in multiple areas. Take the same "lunch with a friend" example and examine the topic of conversation. Are you getting tips on how to get your dog to stop barking all the time? That would add a cognitive layer of learning. Or, are you providing your friend moral support after getting bad news? In that case, your trifecta includes emotional.

Table 6.1 models how a single area of focus can be fed in multiple ways depending on what second area of your wellness it's partnered with. In the first column, each of the five areas of wellness are listed. In each row, the primary activity is modified slightly to include another area of your wellness. Look at the first row labeled "Physical: Go for a walk." In the boxes where physical intersects with emotional, cognitive, social, and spiritual, examples are provided on how a simple walk can double your effort. You can go for a triple by going for a walk with your friend and both of you listening and discussing a podcast. The possibilities are limitless.

You are already experiencing multiplicative wellness. Now that you're mindful of how your self-care contributes to your well-being, you are empowered to make decisions that allow you to be efficient with your choices and layer on areas of your self-care that need attention. If you have been feeling particularly isolated lately, bring someone with you to run errands that you know you need to do anyway.

Strained and drained teachers will find multiplicative wellness to be helpful when it comes to minimizing effort and achieving maximum results. Just remember to include areas that *need* attention as a priority over areas you *want* to tend to.

MATCHING RESPONSES TO ROOT CAUSES

In a 2017 survey conducted by American Federation of Teachers, educators and school staff found their work "always" or "often" stressful a whopping 61 percent of the time. The same scale revealed only 30 percent of general population workers felt the level of stress. Therefore, in order to maintain self-care, it is even more critical that educators build and use coping skills to prevent burnout and avoid the negative consequences stress brings to the body and mind.

Now that you're nearing the end of this book, hopefully you have exposed some areas of your self-care that, if given attention, should make a difference in your wellness. If your list of needs is long, your emotional self might be bubbling up with a feeling of being overwhelmed. When even one area of your self-care is not strong, the impact can be felt in other areas. You aren't getting enough sleep (physical), so you have difficulty concentrating

Table 6.1: Multiplicative Wellness

	Physical	Emotional	Cognitive	Social	Spiritual
Physical Go for a walk.		Take a walk to cool down when you're upset.	Walk and listen to a podcast.	Walk with a friend.	Walk mindfully and take in your connection to nature.
Emotional Take an emotional break.	Turn up the radio and dance!		Play a game that makes you think—but you love!	Cuddle with a loved one.	Meditate and focus on all the things that bring you joy.
Cognitive Learn something new.	Watch YouTube videos on a new exercise style and try it out.	Browse a journal article about how to handle something that makes you anxious.		Interview someone who has a skill you'd like to learn.	Read a few blogs about how to improve in an area where you'd like to personally grow.
Social Spend time with friends.	Go play pickleball, golf, laser tag, or go ice skating.	Reach out to someone you trust when you're down.	Challenge your kids to a game of chess or go to an escape room.		Join a religion study group and meet new people.
Spiritual Label your legacy.	Practice mindful eating to strengthen your ability to focus.	In your gratitude journal, list why others are grateful for YOU.	Create a Pinterest page with examples of how you honor your true self.	Attend a benefit that is raising money for a cause close to your heart.	

(cognitive). An uncomfortable situation is weighing on you (spiritual), causing you to distance yourself from a circle of family or friends (social). You have mounds of paperwork to complete (cognitive) and it's making you impatient with others (emotional and social).

The awareness of how deficits in one area are impacting you in another area is a key to addressing the real needs in your self-care regimen. Let's look at one of the examples in the previous paragraph. You are likely to recognize the symptoms might be contributing to your stress. The inability to concentrate might cause you to take measures to tackle a cognitive need. If your solution is to walk away from your task and give yourself a brain break, you might feel like you're using the strategies you learned in this book. However, if lack of concentration is the effect of only getting five hours of sleep at night, all the brain breaks in the world are not going to address your fuzziness.

Reacting to side effects of inadequate self-care methods is sometimes necessary, but this isn't the most effective way to build a personal wellness program. The approach of waiting for problems to occur and dealing with them as they arise will continue to drain you. Not only does it set you up to continuously feel the strains of life, but how you align your response might not impact the root cause. The result: the stress simmers and flares up repeatedly. The approach of waiting for problems to surface and addressing them when you feel the drain will continue to weigh on your sense of wellness.

To reduce stress, the contributing factors or root causes of stress must be addressed. This requires you to be acutely aware of the true reasons you might be lonely, exhausted, uninspired, or frustrated. Because of the complexities with how areas of wellness overlap, this is more challenging than it sounds. Reflection strategies like journaling, meditation, or working with a professional are some ways to reveal root causes for times when your wellness is suffering. However, it doesn't replace a lifestyle that leads to holistic health. Prevention through continuous attention to self-care, embedded habits, and regular soul searching and reflection will help you assess the state of your physical, emotional, cognitive, social, and spiritual well-being.

SELF-CARE IS THE WAY TO WELLNESS

Self-care is essential for teachers, now more than ever. It can avert feeling strained and drained. Engaging in a self-care routine can help avoid burnout and reduce unhealthy levels of stress (Glowiak, 2020). The reason for filling a metaphorical wellness backpack is to "lighten your load" so you are free to give the attention needed to your job and your life outside of school. The hiking analogy shared in the preface described the benefit of a backpack to free your hands and allow you to use them to teach. When your hands are busy dealing with the result of inadequate self-care practices, they aren't available when you need them, which perpetuates the spiral of stress.

Service professionals such as teachers, find it easier to assume the role of caregiver, rather than take care of themselves (Coaston, 2017). However, when teachers neglect their own needs, every area of their lives suffers. Ongoing high levels of stress impacts your ability to be at your best. The vaccine for strained and drained teachers is a solid self-care system that prevents unhealthy stress levels, develops healthy habits to support your growth, maintains each area of your self-care routines, builds coping skills to address inevitable life challenges, and provides a process for self-assessing the effectiveness of your self-care efforts on your overall wellness.

APPS FOR YOUR WELLNESS BACKPACK

Technology is a valuable contribution to your wellness backpack. Self-care is what you do on a regular basis to support your overall wellness. Apps make it easier to build habits and embed routines of self-care into your life. To get you

Table 6.2: Apps for Your Wellness Backpack

App Name	Key Features
Breathing Zone	Therapeutic breathing exercises, defuses stress, lowers blood pressure
Calm	Meditation, relaxation, mindfulness, breathing techniques, calming exercise, sleep stories
Colorfy	Coloring, painting book, encourages creativity
Couch to 5K	Encourages beginners to run, tracks progress
Day One	Journaling, create entries, optional prompts, ability to customize reminders
Down Dog	Build your own yoga practices, multiple practice types of yoga
Happify	Cheerful quizzes, games, happiness-boosting activities
Headspace	Encourages meditation and mindfulness, themed sessions including sleep, stress, anxiety, and focus
Insight Timer	Yoga, thousands of meditations, sections of sleep, live events, and work
Lumosity	Games for your mind, helps improve memory and problem-solving
NOOM	Personalized weight loss plan, accountability, food calorie counter, pedometer, access to health coach
MapMyRun	Tracks fitness activities, records details of workout and route, interactive map
MyFitnessPal	Log weight, workout, food and fitness goals, online community that you can join for advice, tips, and inspiration
MyPlate	Weight loss, tracks food, logs workouts
Relax Melodies	Sleep sound section sorted into categorizes, encourages you to sleep better
Shine	Mediation, mood tracking, journaling prompts, focuses on mental health
STRAVA	Tracks fitness and exercise, cycling and running emphasis
Streaks	Complete tasks, each day you participate extends your streak
Think Up	Motivation, positive affirmations

started, a list of apps in Table 6.2 is provided. This is not a comprehensive list of all available apps, but will offer you a variety of digital tools to go along with the other strategies you have added to your backpack.

NO REGRETS

Bronnie Ware is an Australian nurse who cared for terminally ill patients in the last twelve weeks of their lives. She wrote about her observations in a blog and then later a book titled *The Top Five Regrets of the Dying* (2012). Ware disclosed the top five regrets patients shared with her. They were:

1. *I wish I had the courage to live a life true to myself, not the life others expected of me*. This was the most common regret.
2. *I wish I had not worked so hard*. Many expressed regret over missing children's youth and companionship time with their partner.
3. *I wish I had the courage to express my feelings*. People often suppress feelings in order to keep peace with others. They settled for a mediocre existence and never became who they felt they were capable of becoming. Many developed illnesses related to the bitterness and resentment they felt.
4. *I wish I had stayed in touch with my friends*. The benefit of old friendships became clear in their last weeks, but they often could not locate the past friends. They were caught up in the busyness of life. There were regrets about not putting the time and effort into friendships.
5. *I wish that I had let myself be happier*. People felt they had stayed stuck in old habits and patterns. They had a fear of change and pretended they were content. Near the end of life, they had an awareness that happiness is a choice.

After working through the exercises in this book, you most likely have a better understanding of what you value. As you continue to focus on yourself as a whole teacher, use strategies in your self-care backpack and center on your core values. Nourish yourself, much like you would need to nourish a plant, and tend to your own needs so you can flourish. Live life according to your true self and do not worry about meeting anyone's expectations but your own. There will always be one more thing to do and demands on your time, but nothing will have a greater impact on your wellness than prioritizing your self-care.

Go back and reread what Ware's patients would have changed in their lives if they could. See if you can identify themes in the regrets these patients realized. They align with the areas of wellness discussed in this book. Spiritual, cognitive, physical, social, and emotional threads can be found in the top five regrets Ware heard. Reflect on what is important in *your* life. Luckily you have time to take action and make the changes now.

AN INVITATION

Your commitment to reading this book is the first step on your journey to developing self-care habits. You are not alone. Many teachers, whether they voice it or not, are feeling overworked and are affected by the strains of teaching. Give your social wellness a bump and invite a colleague to join you in discovering ways to establish a strong self-care system. Write down the names of other teachers who might benefit from reading this book and partnering with you. Not only will you be communicating care and compassion, it could lead to a support system to help you commit to prioritizing your own self-care.

Invitation List

1.
2.
3.
4.
5.

Bibliography

Amen, D. (2012). *Use your brain to change your age: Secrets to look, feel, and think younger every day*. New York: Harmony.

American Federation of Teachers. (2017). Educator quality of work life survey. Retrieved July 1, 2020, from https://www.aft.org/sites/default/files/2017_eqwl_survey_web.pdf

American Psychological Association. (2012). *What you need to know about willpower: The psychological science of self-control*. http://www.apa.org/topics/personality/willpower

American Psychological Association. (2021). One year later, a new wave of pandemic health concerns. Retrieved September 20, 2021, from http://www.apa.org/news/press/releases/stress/2021/one-year-pandemic-stress

Angle, S. (2018). How to Get 150 Minutes of Exercise Each Week. Diabetes Forecast. Retrieved January 22, 2021, from http://www.diabetesforecast.org/2018/05-sep-oct/how-to-get-150-minutes-of.html#:~:text=Research%20from%20the%20University%20of,more%20realistic%2C%E2%80%9D%20says%20Mitchell

Arlinghaus, K. R., & Johnston, C. A. (2018). The importance of creating habits and routine. *American Journal of Lifestyle Medicine, 13*(2), 142–44.

Baumeister, R. F., & Tierney, J. (2011). *Willpower: Rediscovering the greatest human strength*. Penguin Press.

Beaven, C. M., & Ekstrom, J. (2013). A comparison of blue light and caffeine efects on cognitive function and alertness in humans. *PLOS ONE 8*(10). https://doi.org/10.1371/journal.pone.0076707

Better Health Channel. (2018). The dangers of sitting: why sitting is the new smoking. Retrieved January 18, 2021, from https://www.betterhealth.vic.gov.au/health/healthyliving/the-dangers-of-sitting

Bill & Melinda Gates Foundation. (2012). *Primary sources 2012: America's teachers on the teaching profession, a project of Scholastic and the Bill & Melinda Gates Foundation*. Seattle, WA: Author. http://www.scholastic.com/primarysources/pdfs/Gates2012_full.pdf

Blackstock, C. (2011). The emergence of the breath of life theory. *Journal of Social Work Values and Ethics*, *8*(1).

Blackstock, C. (2019). Revisiting the breath of life theory. *British Journal of Social Work, 49*(4), 854–59.

Blanding, M. (2018). Civil actions. *Georgetown Business Magazine*. Retrieved March 22, 2022, from https://msb.georgetown.edu/news-story/civil-actions/

Blood, N., & Heavyhead, R. (2007). Blackfoot influence on Abraham Maslow (Lecture delivered at University of Montana). Blackfoot Digital Library. Retrieved September 29, 2021, from https://www.blackfootdigitallibrary.com/digital/collection/bdl/id/1296/rec/1

Boogren, T. (2018). *Take Time for Your Self-Care: Action Plans for Teachers.* Solution Tree Press.

Bourg-Carter, S. (2013). The tell tale signs of burnout. Do you aave them? *Psychology Today*. https://www.psychologytoday.com/us/blog/high-octane-women/201311/the-tell-tale-signs-burnout-do-you-have-them

Bradberry, T. (2016). 6 toxic relationships you should avoid like the plague. TalentSmarteq. Retrieved September 24, 2021, from https://www.talentsmarteq.com/articles/6-Toxic-Relationships-You-Should-Avoid-Like-the-Plague-586622299-p-1.html/

Bratman, G. N., Dailey, C. D., Levy, B. J. & Gross, J. J. (2015). The benefits of nature experience: Improved affect and cognition. *Landscape and Urban Planning, 138,* 41–45.

Brooks, S., & Joseph, M. X. (2019). *Modern mentor: Reimagining mentorship in education*. Times 10 Publications.

Brown, B. (2010). *The gifts of imperfection: Let go of who you think you're* supposed *to be and embrace who you are*. Hazelden Publishing.

Brown, B. (2015). *Rising strong*. Vermilion.

Brown, B. (2018). *Dare to lead.* Vermilion.

Brown, M.. & Bussell, J. (2011). Medication adherence: WHO cares? *Mayo Clinic Proceedings, 86*(4), 304–14.

Burgess, L. (2017). Eight benefits of crying: Why it's good to shed a few tears. Medical News Today. Retrieved August 28, 2021, from https://www.medicalnewstoday.com/articles/319631

Cain, S. (2013). *Quiet: The power of introverts in a world that can't stop talking.* Broadway Books.

Campbell, S. (2015). The happiness doctor is in. Next Avenue. Retrieved September 30, 2021, from https://www.nextavenue.org/the-happiness-doctor-is-in/

Centofanti, S., Banks, S., Coussens, S., Gray, D., Munro, E., Nielsen, J., & Dorrian, J. (2020). A pilot study investigating the impact of a caffeine-nap on alertness during a simulated night shift. *Chronobiology International*, *37*(9–10), 1469–73. DOI: 10.1080/07420528.2020.1804922

Cherry, K. (2020). How to improve your self-control. Very Well Mind. Retrieved on August 2, 2021, from https://www.verywellmind.com/psychology-of-self-control-4177125

Coaston, S. (2017). Self-care through self-compassion: A balm for burnout. *The Professional Counselor, 7*(3), 285–97.

Coffeng, J., Sluijs, E., Hendriksen, I., Mechelen, W., & Boot, C. (2015). Physical activity and relaxation during and after work are independently associated with the need for recovery. *Journal of Physical Activity and Health, 12*(1), 109–15.

Cohen, S., Janicki-Deverts, D., Turner, R. B., & Doyle, W. J. (2015). Does hugging provide stress-buffering social support? A study of susceptibility to upper respiratory infection and illness. *Psychological Science, 26*(2), 135–147.

Coleman, J. (2016). Why business people should join book clubs. *Harvard Business Review*. Retrieved January 10, 2021, from https://hbr.org/2016/02/why-businesspeople-should-join-book-clubs

Constantinou, E., Van Den Houte, M., Bogaerts, K., Van Diest, I.. & Van den Bergh, O. (2014). Can words heal? Using affect labeling to reduce the effects of unpleasant cues on symptom reporting. *Frontiers in Psychology, 5*, Article 807.

Coughlan, S. (2016). UN says 69 million teachers needed for global school pledge. BBC News. Retrieved September 28, 2021, from https://www.bbc.com/news/business-37544983

Covey, S. R. (1989). *The seven habits of highly effective people: Restoring the character ethic*. Simon and Schuster.

Critcher, C. R., & Dunning, D. (2015). Self-affirmations provide a broader perspective on self-threat. *Personality and Social Psychology Bulletin, 41*(1), 3–18.

Csikszentmihalyi, M. (1990). *Flow: The psychology of optimal experience*. Harper and Row.

DeFrance, K. (2020). The power of emotion mindsets. *Psychology Today*. Retrieved August 28, 2021, from https://www.psychologytoday.com/us/blog/the-science-feeling/202010/the-power-emotion-mindsets

Dimitriu, A. (2020). Circadian rhythm. Sleep Foundation. Retrieved January 16, 2021, from https://www.sleepfoundation.org/circadian-rhythm

Dodgson, L. (2018). What everyone gets wrong about introverts—including why they are not antisocial or lazy. Retrieved on August 28, 2021, from https://www.businessinsider.com/what-its-like-to-be-an-introvert-and-what-everyone-gets-wrong-2018-5

Ducharme, J. (2019). Why spending time with friends is one of the best things you can do for your health. *Time*. Retrived from https://time.com/5609508/social-support-health-benefits/

Ducrot P., Méjean, C., Aroumougame, V., et al. (2017). Meal planning is associated with food variety, diet quality and body weight status in a large sample of French adults. *International Journal of Behavioral Nutrition and Physical Activity, 14*(1),12.

Duvivier, B., Schaper, N., Bremers, M., van Crombrugge, G., Menheere, P., Kars, M., & Savelberg, H. (2013). Minimal intensity physical activity (standing and walking) of longer duration improves insulin action and plasma lipids more than shorter periods of moderate to vigorous exercise (cycling) in sedentary subjects when energy expenditure is comparable. *PLoS One, 8*(2), e55542.

Dweck, C. S. (2006). *Mindset: The new psychology of success*. New York: Random House.

Eilam, D., Izhar, R., & Mort, J. (2011). Threat detection: Behavioral practices in animals and humans. *Neuroscience and Biobehavioral Reviews, 35*(4), 999–1006.

Emmonds, R. (2010). Why gratitude is good. *Greater Good Magazine*. Retrieved August 28, 2021, from https://greatergood.berkeley.edu/article/item/why_gratitude_is_good

Emotion wheel chart. (2021, May 10). The Junto Institute. https://www.thejuntoinstitute.com/emotion-wheels/

Galderisi, S., Heinz, A., Kastrup, M., Beezhold, J., & Sartorius, N. (2015). Toward a new definition of mental health. *World Psychiatry, 14*(2), 231–33.

Global Wellness Institute. (2021, September 3). What is wellness? https://globalwellnessinstitute.org/what-is-wellness/

Glowiak, M. (2020). What is self-care and why is it important for you? South New Hampshire University. Retrieved July 15, 2021, from https://www.snhu.edu/about-us/newsroom/health/what-is-self-care

Gobin, R. (2019). *The self care prescription: Powerful solutions to manage stress, reduce anxiety and increase* well-being. Althea Press.

Godfrey, C. M., Harrison, M. B., Lysaght R., Lamb M., Graham, I. D., & Oakley, P. (2010). The experience of self-care: A systematic review. *JBI Library of Systematic Reviews, 8*(34), 1351–1460.

Gracanin, A. Bylsma, L., & Vingerhoets, J. (2014). Is crying a self-soothing behavior ? *Frontiers in Psychology, 5,* 502. https://doi.org/10.3389/fpsyg.2014.00502

Greenberg, M., Brown, J., & Abenavoli, R. (2016). *Teacher stress and health effects of teachers, students, and schools*. Pennsylvania State University.

Greger, M. (2015). *How not to die: Discover the foods scientifically proven to prevent and reverse disease*. Flatiron Books.

Hariri, A. R., Bookheimer, S. Y., & Mazziotta, J. C. (2000). Modulating emotional responses: Effects of a neocortical network on the limbic system. *Neuroreport, 11*(1), 43–48.

Harris, P. R., & Epton, T. (2009). The impact of self-affirmation on health cognition, health behaviour and other health-related responses: A narrative review. *Social and Personality Psychology Compass, 3*(6), 962–78.

Hartanto, A., Quek, F., Tng, G., & Yong, J. C. (2021). Does social media use increase depressive symptoms? A reverse causation perspective. *Frontiers in Psychiatry*. Retrieved March 2, 2022, from https://www.frontiersin.org/articles/10.3389/fpsyt.2021.641934/full

Harvard Health Letter. (2020). Blue light has a dark side. Retrieved January 16, 2021, from https://www.health.harvard.edu/staying-healthy/blue-light-has-a-dark-side

Heide, M. (2013). Are you really drinking enough water? *ABC News*. Retrieved March 21, 2022, from https://abcnews.go.com/Health/drinking-water/story?id=21213931

Herman, K., Hickmon-Rosa, J., & Reinke, W. (2018). Empirically derived profiles of teacher stress, burnout, self-efficacy, and coping and associated student outcomes. *Journal of Positive Behavior Interventions*, *20*(2), 90–100.

Hess, A. (2021). I felt like I was being experimented on: 1 in 4 teachers are considering quitting after this past year. CNBC News. Retrieved August 27, 2021, from https://www.cnbc.com/2021/06/24/1-in-4-teachers-are-considering-quitting-after-this-past-year.html

Holt-Lunstad, J., Smith, T. B., & Layton, J. B. (2010). Social relationships and mortality risk: A meta-analytic review. *PLoS Medicine*, 7(7). https://doi.org/10.1371/journal.pmed.1000316

Horne, J., Anderson, C., & Platen, C. (2008). Sleep extension versus nap or coffee, within the context of sleep debt. *Journal of Sleep Research, 17*(4), 432–36.

Hotta, K., Kamiya, K., Shimizu, R., Yokoyama, M., Nakamura-Ogura, M., Tabata, M., Kamekawa, D., Akiyama, A., Kato, M., Noda, C., Matsunaga, A., & Masuda, T. (2013). Stretching exercises enhance vascular endothelial function and improve peripheral circulation in patients with acute myocardial infarction. *International Heart Journal 54*(2), 59–63.

Houston, E. (2021). Introvert vs. extrovert: A look at the spectrum and psychology. Positive Psychology. Retrieved September 24, 2021, from https://positivepsychology.com/introversion-extroversion-spectrum/

Iberlin, J. M. (2017). *Cultivating mindfulness in the classroom*. Marzano Resources.

Jahns, L. Savis-Shaw, W., Lichtenstein, A., Murphy, S., Conrad, Z., & Nielsen, F. (2018). The history and future of dietary guidance in America. *Advances in Nutrition, 9*(2), 136–47.

Jensen, E. (2001). *Arts with the brain in mind*. Association for the Supervision of Curriculum Development.

Kaufman, S. B. (2019). Who created Maslow's iconic pyramid? *Scientific American*. Retrieved on September 29, 2021, from https://blogs.scientificamerican.com/beautiful-minds/who-created-maslows-iconic-pyramid/

Kebede, A., Abebe, S., Woldie, H., & Yenit, M. (2019). Low back pain associated factors among primary school teachers in Mekele City, North Ethiopia: A cross-sectional study. *Occupational Therapy International*. https://doi.org/10.1155/2019/3862946

Killingsworth, M., & Gilbert, D. (2010). Wandering mind, not a happy mind. *Harvard Gazette*. Retrieved on September 9, 2021, from https://news.harvard.edu/gazette/story/2010/11/wandering-mind-not-a-happy-mind/

Klemm, W. (2016). Organize for better thinking and memory. *Psychology Today*. Retrieved May 18, 2021, from https://www.psychologytoday.com/us/blog/memory-medic/201604/organize-better-thinking-and-memory

Kotler, J. (2017). Want a Happier work atmosphere? Science says to follow these 10 tips. Inc. Retrieved January 11, 2021, from https://www.inc.com/john-rampton/what-makes-people-happy-when-they-work.html

Krantz-Kent, R. (2008). Teachers' work patterns: when, where, and how much do U.S. teachers work? *Monthly Labor Review, 131*(3), 52.

Laskowski, E. (2021). How much should the average adult exercise every day ? Mayo Clinic. Retrieved January 21, 2021, from https://www.mayoclinic.org/healthy-lifestyle/fitness/expert-answers/exercise/faq-20057916#:~:text=Get%20at%20least%20150%20minutes,provide%20even%20greater%20health%20benefit

Lathrap, Mary. (1895). *The poems and written addresses of Mary T. Lathrap . . . with a short sketch of her life*. Bay City: Woman's Christian Temperance Union of Michigan.

Lee, C. (2017). The science behind the world's most popular drug. McGill Office for Science and Society. Retrieved January 17, 2021, from https://www.mcgill.ca/oss/article/infographics-general-science/science-behind-worlds-most-popular-drug

Lee, I., Shiroma, E., Kamada, M., Bassett, D., Matthews, C., & Buring, J. (2019). Association of step volume and intensity with all-cause mortality in older women. *JAMA Internal Medicine, 179*(8), 1105–12.

Lieberman, M.D., Inagaki, T.K., Tabibnia, G. & Crockett, M.J. (2011). Subjective responses to emotional stimuli during labeling, reappraisal, and distraction. *Emotion, 11*(3), 468–80.

Lin, S., Faust, L., Robles-Granda, P., Kajdanowicz, T., & Chawla, N. (2019). Social network structure is predictive of health and wellness. *PLOS ONE 14*(6), e0217264. https://doi.org/10.1371/journal.pone.0217264

Lino, C. (2020). The psychology of willpower: Training the brain for better decisions. Positive Psychology. Retrieved January 17, 2021, from https://positivepsychology.com/psychology-of-willpower/

Lou, E., & Watson, K. (2019). How Long Can You Go Without Peeing? Healthline. Retrieved January 16, 2021, from https://www.healthline.com/health/how-long-can-you-go-without-peeing

Lynch, S. (2017). How to deal with toxic people at work. *Greater Good Magazine*. Retrieved September 24, 2021, from https://greatergood.berkeley.edu/article/item/how_to_deal_with_toxic_people_at_work

Manella, M. (2016). Study: A third of U.S. adults don't get enough sleep. Retrieved on March 21, 2022, from https://www.cnn.com/2016/02/18/health/one-third-americans-dont-sleep-enough/index.html

Marcin, A. (2019). How much water you need to drink. Healthline. Retrieved January 22, 2021, from https://www.healthline.com/health/how-much-water-should-I-drink

Marengo, K. (2018). How long does caffeine stay in your system? *Healthline*. Retrieved March 21, 2022, from https://www.healthline.com/health/how-long-does-caffeine-last#how-long-symptoms-last

Maslow, A. H. (1969). The farther reaches of human nature. *Journal of Transpersonal Psychology, 1*(1), 1–9.

Matthews, G. (2015). Goals Research Summary. Paper presented at the 9th Annual International Conference of the Psychology Research Unit of Athens Institute for Education and Research (ATINER), Athens, Greece.

Mayo Clinic Staff. (2020). Napping: Do's and don'ts for healthy adults. Mayo Clinic. Retrieved August 3, 2021, from https://www.mayoclinic.org/healthy-lifestyle/adult-health/in-depth/napping/art-20048319

McMains, S., & Kastner, S. (2011). Interactions of top-down and bottom-up mechanisms in human visual cortex. *Journal of Neuroscience 31*(2), 587–97. https://doi.org/10.1523/JNEUROSCI.3766-10.2011

Michel, K. L. (2014). Maslow's hierarchy connected to Blackfoot beliefs. *Karen Lincoln Michel blog*. Retrieved from https://lincolnmichel.wordpress.com/2014/04/19/maslows-hierarchy-connected-to-blackfoot-beliefs/

Miller, A. (2017). The science behind the case for routines. *Parent*. Retrieved January 11, 2021, from https://www.parent.com/the-science-behind-the-case-for-routines/

Miller, J., & Lambert, V. (2018). *Boundaries*. Harlequin HQN.

Moore, C. (2021). Positive daily affirmations: Is there science behind it? Positive Psychology. Retrieved August 28, 2021, from https://positivepsychology.com/daily-affirmations/

National Network of Depression Centers. *Get the facts*. Retrieved March 16, 2022, from https://nndc.org/facts/

National Sleep Foundation 2013 poll. Retrieved March 21, 2022, from https://www.sleepfoundation.org/professionals/sleep-america-polls

Nelson, M. (2013, September 13). How to drink more water each day. *U.S. News & World Report*. https://health.usnews.com/health-news/blogs/eat-run/2013/09/13/how-to-drink-more-water-each-day#:~:text=Two%20hours%20prior%20to%20exercise%2C%20drink%2017%20to%2020%20ounces.&text=Every%2010%20to%2020%20minutes,drink%207%20to%2010%20ounces.&text=Following%20exercise%20(whether%20you're,pound%20of%20body%20weight%20loss.

Ni, Y. & Rorrer, A. K. (2018). *Why do teachers choose teaching and remain teaching: Initial results from the Educator Career and Pathway Survey (ECAPS) for teachers*. Utah Education Policy Center.

Nichols, H. (2018). Why you feel tired all the time. Medical News Today. Retrieved August 8, 2021, from https://www.medicalnewstoday.com/articles/320800

Owens, S. J. (2015). *Georgia's teacher dropout crisis: A look at why nearly half of Georgia public school teachers are leaving the profession*. Georgia Department of Education. Retrieved September 27, 2021, from www.gadoe.org/External-Affairs-and-Policy/communications/Documents/Teacher%20Survey%20Results.pdf

Parr, C. (2021). Tes focus on . . . skipping lunch at school. *Tes Magazine*. Retrieved March 22, 2022, from https://www.tes.com/magazine/teaching-learning/general/tes-focus-onskipping-lunch-school

Pew Research Center. (2021). Measuring religion in Pew Research Center's American Trends Panel. Retrieved September 30, 2021, from https://www.pewforum.org/2021/01/14/measuring-religion-in-pew-research-centers-american-trends-panel/

Phelan, H. (2018, October 25). What's all this about journaling? *New York Times*. https://www.nytimes.com/2018/10/25/style/journaling-benefits.html

Piercy, K., & Troiano, R. (2018). Physical activity guidelines for Americans from the United States Department of Health and Human Services. *Cardiovascular Quality and Outcomes, 11*(11). Retrieved from https://doi.org/10.1161/CIRCOUTCOMES.118.005263

Piercy, K. L., Troiano, R. P., Ballard, R. M., Carlson, S. A., Fulton, J.E., Galuska, D. A., George S. M., & Olson R. D. (2018). The physical activity guidelines for Americans. *JAMA 320*(19), 2020–28.

Porath, D. (2016). An antidote to incivility. *Harvard Business Review*. Retrieved August 28, 2021, from https://hbr.org/2016/04/an-antidote-to-incivility

Rakal, D. (2016). Learning deep breathing. Psych Central. Retrieved January 17, 2021, from https://psychcentral.com/lib/learning-deep-breathing#1

Rampton, J. (2017). Want a happier work atmosphere? Science says to follow these 10 tips. Inc. Retrieved January 10, 2021, https://www.inc.com/john-rampton/what-makes-people-happy-when-they-work.html

Ravilochan, T. (2021). What I got wrong: Revisions to my post about the Blackfoot and Maslow. GatherFor. Retrieved September 29, 2021, from https://gatherfor.medium.com/i-got-it-wrong-7d9b314fadff

Raypole, C. (2020). Let it out: Dealing with repressed emotions. Healthline. Retrieved August 8, 2021, from https://www.healthline.com/health/repressed-emotions

Reading Agency. (2015). Literature review: The impact of reading for pleasure and empowerment. *BOP Consulting*. Retrieved March 21, 2022, from https://readingagency.org.uk/news/The%20Impact%20of%20Reading%20for%20Pleasure%20and%20Empowerment.pdf

Remmers, C., Topolinski, S., & Koole, S. (2016). Why being mindful may have more benefits than you realize: Mindfulness improves both explicit and implicit mood regulation. *Mindfulness 7,* 829–37.

Sackstein, S., & Hamilton, C. (2016). *Hacking homework: 10 strategies that inspire learning outside the classroom*. Cleveland, OH: X10 Publications.

Santos-Longhurst, A. (2018). How to treat and prevent mental exhaustion. Healthline. Retrieved on January 11, 2021, on https://www.healthline.com/health/mental-exhaustion

Santos-Longhurst, A. (2019). What are the benefits of kickboxing? Healthline. Retrieved August 28, 2021, https://www.healthline.com/health/kickboxing-benefitsfrom

Schweitzer, P. K., Randazzo, A. C., Stone K., Erman, M., & Walsh, J. K. (2006). Laboratory and field studies of naps and caffeine as practical countermeasures for sleep-wake problems associated with night work. *Sleep, 29*(1), 39–50. doi: 10.1093/sleep/29.1.39. PMID: 16453980.

Scott, E. (2020a). The Overwhelming Benefits of Power Napping. VeryWellMind. Retrieved on January, 21 from https://www.verywellmind.com/power-napping-health-benefits-and-tips-stress-3144702

Scott, E. (2020b). Why Self Care Can Help You Manage Stress. VeryWellMind. Retrieved on January 20, 2021, from https://www.verywellmind.com/importance-of-self-care-for-health-stress-management-3144704#:~:text=May%20Boost%20Physical%20Health,stress%20from%20damaging%20your%20health

Scutti, S. (2017). Yes, sitting too long can kill you even if you exercise. *CNN*. Retrieved March 21, 2022, from https://www.cnn.com/2017/09/11/health/sitting-increases-risk-of-death-study/index.html

Silverman, A., Logel, C., & Cohen, G. (2013). Self-affirmation as a deliberate coping strategy: The moderating role of choice. *Journal of Experimental Social Psychology, 49*(1), 93–98.

Smith, Z. (2019). 5 advantages of getting fresh air. Thrive Global. Retrieved January 16, 2021, from https://thriveglobal.com/stories/5-advantages-of-getting-fresh-air/

Sparks, D. (2019). Mayo mindfulness: Connecting spirituality and stress relief. *Mayo Clinic News Network*. Retrieved March 22, 2022, from https://newsnetwork.mayoclinic.org/discussion/mayo-mindfulness-connecting-spirituality-and-stress-relief/

Spector, N. (2017). Smiling can trick your brain into happiness—and boost your health. Better by Today. Retrieved August 28, 2021, from https://www.nbcnews.com/better/health/smiling-can-trick-your-brain-happiness-boost-your-health-ncna822591

Stanborough, R. (2019). Benefits of reading books: How it Can positively affect your life. *Healthline*. Retrieved March 21, 2022, from https://www.healthline.com/health/benefits-of-reading-books#takeaway

Suni, E. (2020). How to determine poor sleep quality. Sleep Foundation. Retrieved January 17, 2021, from_https://www.sleepfoundation.org/sleep-hygiene/how-to-determine-poor-quality-sleep

Suttie, J. (2017). How smartphones are killing conversation. *Greater Good Magazine*. Retrieved September 25, 2021, from https://greatergood.berkeley.edu/article/item/how_smartphones_are_killing_conversation

Taylor, N. & Millear, P. (2016). The contribution of mindfulness to predicting burnout in the workplace. *Personality and Individual Differences*, *89*, 123–28.

Terkeurst, L. (2018). *It's not supposed to be this way: Finding unexpected strength when disappointments leave you shattered.* Thomas Nelson.

Trust, T., Krutka, D., & Carpenter, J. (2016). Together we are better: Professional learning networks for teachers. *Computers & Education, 102*, 15–34.

Tunikova, O. (2018). The science of willpower: How to train your productivity muscle. Medium. Retrieved January 17, 2021, from https://medium.com/@tunikova_k/the-science-of-willpower-how-to-train-your-productivity-muscle-8b2738ce745b

United States Department of Agriculture. (2021). What foods are included in the dairy group? MyPlate.gov. Retrieved September 29, 2021, from https://www.myplate.gov/eat-healthy/dairy

United States Department of Health and Human Services. (2018). *Physical activity guidelines for Americans, 2nd edition.* Washington, DC: Author.

University of Missouri-Columbia. (2020). Teacher stress linked with higher risk of student suspensions: Study examines impact of teacher burnout on student behavior, discipline issues. ScienceDaily. www.sciencedaily.com/releases/2020/09/200915105929.htm.

University of Texas at Austin. (2011). Psychologists find the meaning of aggression: "Monty Python" scene helps research. ScienceDaily. Retrieved September 21, 2021, from www.sciencedaily.com/releases/2011/03/110323105202.htm.

Vora, P. (2015). Nearly half of American adults clueless about their annual health check-up. *Pharmacy Times*. Retrieved March 22, 2022, from https://www.pharmacytimes.com/view/nearly-half-of-american-adults-clueless-about-their-annual-health-check-up

Walsh, B. (2017, August 7). Does spirituality make you happy? *Time*. https://time.com/4856978/spirituality-religion-happiness/

Ware, B. (2012). *The top five regrets of dying: A life transformed by the dearly departing*. Hay House.

Weir, K. (2011). The exercise effect. *American Psychological Association, 42*(11), 48.

Wheelwright, T. (2021). Cell phone behavior in 2021: How obsessed are we? Reviews.org. Retrieved September 29, 2021, from https://www.reviews.org/mobile/cell-phone-addiction/#:~:text=re%20not%20alone.-,On%20average%2C%20Americans%20check%20their%20phones%20262%20times%20per%20day,that%27s%20once%20every%205.5%20minutes

About the Authors

Connie Hamilton, EdS, is a dedicated educator and mother of three grown children. In her 20+ years working in schools, she has served the profession as a teacher, instructional coach, principal, and district curriculum director. As a principal, she was honored as the Ionia County Service Learning Administrator of the Year. In her leadership roles, Connie has been part of wellness planning for her district's staff. She secured grant funds to provide healthy foods for students and their families during school-sponsored social events. Connie was the recipient of the Service Learning Administrator of the Year. As principal, she worked collaboratively with food service to schedule breakfast options that allow for on-time start of the school day and implement wellness policies that impacted school lunch menus, classroom snacks, and school rewards. Connie was also awarded a grant that provided funds for the school social worker to initiate a Girls on the Run program in her elementary school. Her experience with cognitive behavior therapy has not only provided her with de-escalation strategies in intense moments but has given her the opportunity to share tools with others to support children and adults with anxiety.

Currently, Connie works directly with teachers in intimate settings to support their professional growth. She is the author of two books, *Hacking Homework: 10 Strategies That Inspire Learning Outside the Classroom* (2016) and *Hacking Questions: 11 Answers That Create a Culture of Inquiry in Your Classroom* (2019). Her focus on the whole teacher sets her apart to build trust and establish rapport with educators. Connie's dynamic presentation style is applauded by her audiences. Tangible strategies that are supported by research empower and motivate teachers to use the learning they gained by attending one of her workshops. Referred to as the "Questioning Guru," Connie has a unique ability to coach educators to guide them through reflection and professional discovery in a way that brings out the best in them.

Dorothy VanderJagt, EdD, is a popular and engaging speaker who works with educators all over the country in supporting professional practices and igniting learning. She is the author of *Permission to Pause: A Journal for*

Teachers (2020), *Zip-Around Direction Games: Ready-to-use, Interactive Activities to Practice Reading and Active Listening* (2009), *Zip-Around Math Games: Ready-to-use, Interactive Activities to Practice Problem Solving* (2009), as well as co-author of *Fire Up for Learning: Active Learning Projects and Activities to Motivate and Challenge Students* (2002) and *Wow, What a Team! Essential Components for Successful Teaming* (2001). Dorothy is an award-winning educator and has over thirty years in the profession as a teacher and leader. She was a teacher for ten years, a principal for eleven years, and a curriculum director for four years. Dorothy served as a leader on her district's wellness team.

Dorothy currently serves as a coordinator for the High Impact Leadership Project which supports 150 schools with literacy and leadership and is the director of the Michigan Education Conference. Dorothy teaches graduate courses and has published research on problems facing schools today, leadership, curriculum strategies, and self-care. Dorothy is the founder and president of iFireUP, a premier provider of conferences and online learning. She is known for developing energizing, educational workshops that provide educators with practical strategies for immediate use.

Made in the USA
Columbia, SC
27 August 2024